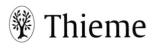

Pocket Atlas of Sectional Anatomy

Computed Tomography and Magnetic Resonance Imaging

Volume I
Head and Neck

Torsten B. Moeller, MD
Department of Radiology
Caritas Hospital
Dillingen, Germany

Emil Reif, MD
Department of Radiology
Caritas Hospital
Dillingen, Germany

Third edition, revised and updated

413 illustrations

Thieme
Stuttgart · New York

Library of Congress Cataloging-in-Publication Data is available from the publisher.

This book is an authorized and revised translation of the German 3rd edition published and copyrighted 2005 by Georg Thieme Verlag, Stuttgart, Germany. Title of the German edition: Taschenatlas der Schnittbildanatomie. Computertomographie und Kernspintomographie. Band I: Kopf, Hals

Translator: Barbara Herzberger, MD, Munich, Germany
Illustrator: Barbara Gay, Stuttgart, Germany

1st German edition 1993
1st English edition 1994
1st Japanese edition 1994
1st Greek edition 1995
1st Spanish edition 1995
1st German edition 1997
1st French edition 1999
2nd English edition 2000
2nd Japanese edition 2000
2nd French edition 2001
2nd Spanish edition 2001
2nd Greek edition 2002
1st Portuguese edition (for Brazil) 2002
3rd German edition 2005

© 2007 Georg Thieme Verlag KG
Rüdigerstraße 14,
70469 Stuttgart, Germany
http://www.thieme.de
Thieme New York, 333 Seventh Avenue,
New York, NY 10001, USA
http://www.thieme.com

Cover design: Thieme Verlagsgruppe
Typesetting by primustype R. Hurler GmbH, 73274 Notzingen
Printed in Germany by Appl Aprinta Druck, Wemding

ISBN 10: 3-13-125503-x (GTV)
ISBN 13: 978-3-13-125503-7 (GTV)
ISBN 10: 1-58890-475-x (TNY)
ISBN 13: 978-1-58890-475-1 (TNY)
      1 2 3 4 5 6

Important note: Medicine is an ever-changing science undergoing continual development. Research and clinical experience are continually expanding our knowledge, in particular our knowledge of proper treatment and drug therapy. Insofar as this book mentions any dosage or application, readers may rest assured that the authors, editors, and publishers have made every effort to ensure that such references are in accordance with **the state of knowledge at the time of production of the book.**
Nevertheless, this does not involve, imply, or express any guarantee or responsibility on the part of the publishers in respect to any dosage instructions and forms of applications stated in the book. **Every user is requested to examine carefully** the manufacturers' leaflets accompanying each drug and to check, if necessary in consultation with a physician or specialist, whether the dosage schedules mentioned therein or the contraindications stated by the manufacturers differ from the statements made in the present book. Such examination is particularly important with drugs that are either rarely used or have been newly released on the market. Every dosage schedule or every form of application used is entirely at the user's own risk and responsibility. The authors and publishers request every user to report to the publishers any discrepancies or inaccuracies noticed. If errors in this work are found after publication, errata will be posted at www.thieme.com on the product description page. Some of the product names, patents, and registered designs referred to in this book are in fact registered trademarks or proprietary names even though specific reference to this fact is not always made in the text. Therefore, the appearance of a name without designation as proprietary is not to be construed as a representation by the publisher that it is in the public domain.

Dedicated in love and gratitude
to our parents,
Alfred and Friedel Moeller and
Emil and Edith Reif.

Preface

This book presents the basic anatomy needed to interpret modern sectional images.

In making a diagnosis from sectional images, even experienced diagnosticians must adapt their thinking to the sectional portrayal of anatomic features. The *Pocket Atlas of Sectional Anatomy* aims to facilitate this process by presenting the two modalities that have the greatest practical importance in modern sectional imaging: computed tomography and magnetic resonance imaging.

The importance of these modalities rests partly on their high resolution. So many of the images were produced with 3-tesla instruments. We wish to express our gratitude to the manufacturers, Siemens and Philips.

We have attempted to provide vivid, comprehensive coverage of sectional anatomic details while still making the book compact and easy to use. The four-color illustrations were considered an essential part of this goal to maintain clarity despite the quantity of information.

The contents of the three volumes (I: Head and Neck, II: Chest and Abdomen, and III: Musculoskeletal System), which comprise a unit, follow a strict format in which each CT or MR image is accompanied by a correlative color diagram and a reduced-scale schematic drawing indicating the level of the section. This format conveys maximum information in a minimum of space.

All the images were obtained in patients or volunteers. We wish to express our special gratitude for the production of the images to our radiolologic technologists, Monika Baumann, Silke Koehl, Sabine Mattil, Stefanie Mueller, Heike Philippi, Brigitte Schild, and Petra Weber, as well as to Birgit Reuter and Marion Hellinger from the Siemens manufacturing center. We sincerely thank our fellow physicians, Nadine Dillinger, Heike Ringling, Sigrid Roth, and especially Simone Zenner, for their helpful discussions and suggestions.

Torsten B. Moeller
Emil Reif

Contents

Cranial CT

Cranial MRI

Neck

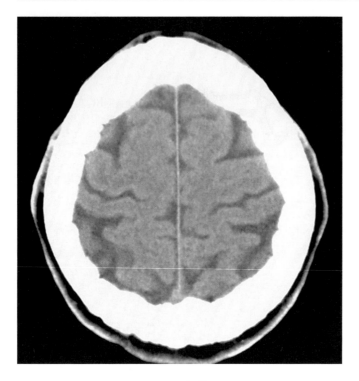

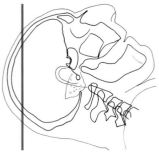

Frontal lobe
Parietal lobe

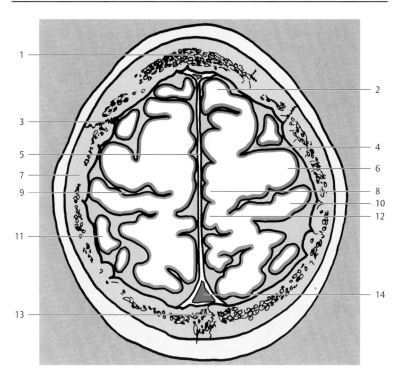

1   Frontal bone
2   Superior frontal gyrus
3   Coronal suture
4   Precentral sulcus
5   Falx cerebri
6   Precentral gyrus
7   Parietal bone
8   Paracentral lobule
9   Central sulcus
10 Postcentral gyrus
11 Superior parietal lobule
12 Precuneus
13 Sagittal suture
14 Superior sagittal sinus

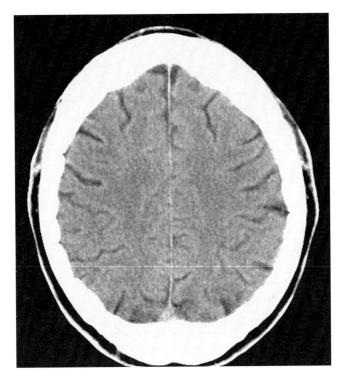

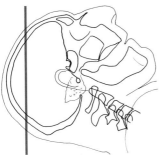

Frontal lobe
Parietal lobe

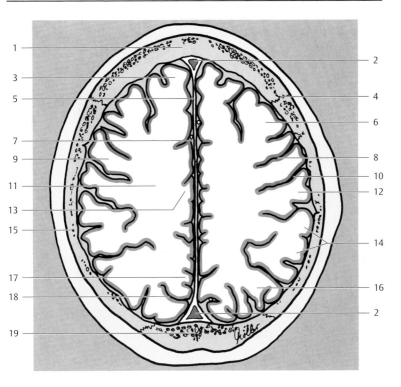

1 Frontal bone
2 Superior sagittal sinus
3 Superior frontal gyrus
4 Coronal suture
5 Falx cerebri
6 Middle frontal gyrus
7 Longitudinal cerebral fissure
8 Precentral sulcus
9 Precentral gyrus
10 Central sulcus
11 Cerebral white matter
   (semioval center)
12 Postcentral gyrus
13 Paracentral lobule
14 Supramarginal gyrus
15 Parietal bone
16 Inferior parietal lobule
17 Precuneus
18 Parieto-occipital sulcus
19 Occipital bone

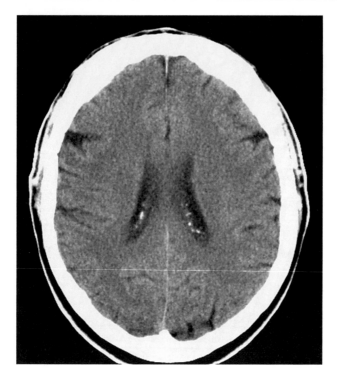

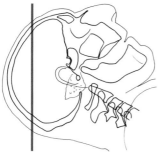

■ Frontal lobe
■ Parietal lobe
■ Occipital lobe

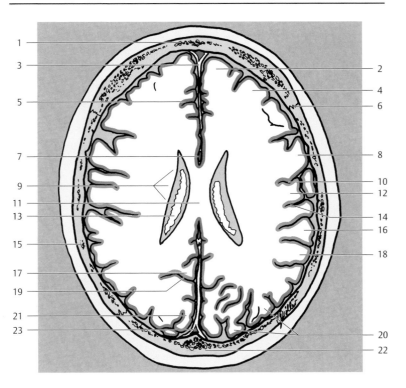

1 Frontal bone
2 Superior frontal gyrus
3 Falx cerebri
4 Middle frontal gyrus
5 Cingulate sulcus
6 Coronal suture
7 Pericallosal
   artery
8 Precentral gyrus
9 Corona radiata
10 Central sulcus
11 Corpus callosum
12 Postcentral gyrus
13 Lateral ventricle (choroid plexus)
14 Postcentral sulcus
15 Parietal bone
16 Supramarginal gyrus
17 Precuneus
18 Angular gyrus
19 Parieto-occipital sulcus
20 Occipital gyri
21 Cuneus
22 Occipital bone
23 Superior sagittal sinus

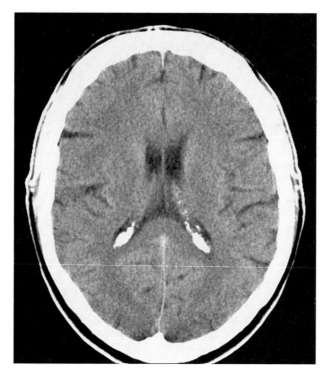

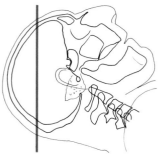

Frontal lobe
Temporal lobe
Parietal lobe
Occipital lobe

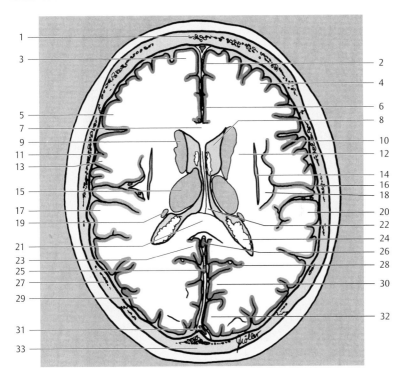

1 Frontal bone
2 Falx cerebri
3 Superior frontal gyrus
4 Middle frontal gyrus
5 Inferior frontal gyrus
6 Cingulate gyrus
7 Corpus callosum (trunk)
8 Lateral ventricle (anterior horn)
9 Caudate nucleus (head)
10 Precentral gyrus
11 Central sulcus
12 Corona radiata
13 Postcentral gyrus
14 Claustrum
15 Thalamus
16 Lateral sulcus
17 Temporal operculum
18 Insula
19 Caudate nucleus (tail)
20 Superior temporal gyrus
21 Corpus callosum (splenium)
22 Fornix
23 Cingulum
24 Lateral ventricle (collateral trigone, choroid plexus)
25 Straight sinus
26 Great cerebral vein (vein of Galen)
27 Parietal bone
28 Parieto-occipital sulcus
29 Occipital gyri
30 Cuneus
31 Superior sagittal sinus
32 Striate cortex
33 Occipital bone

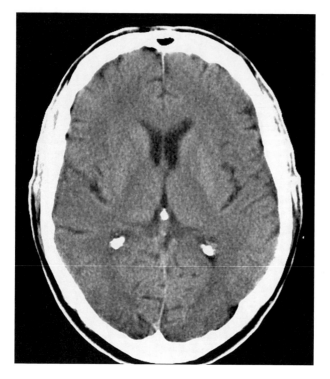

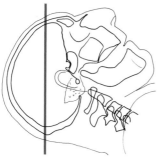

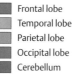

Frontal lobe
Temporal lobe
Parietal lobe
Occipital lobe
Cerebellum

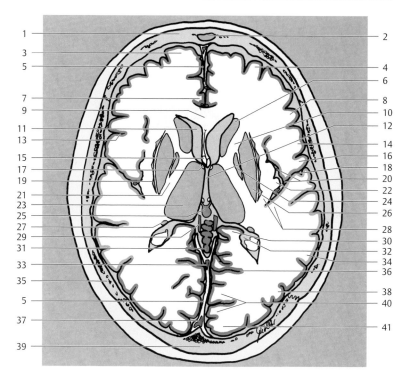

1 Frontal bone
2 Frontal sinus
3 Superior frontal gyrus
4 Middle frontal gyrus
5 Falx cerebri
6 Caudate nucleus (head)
7 Cingulate gyrus
8 Inferior frontal gyrus
9 Corpus callosum (genu)
10 Internal capsule (anterior limb)
11 Lateral ventricle (anterior horn)
12 Third ventricle
13 Central sulcus
14 Precentral gyrus
15 Fornix
16 Postcentral gyrus
17 Interventricular foramen (foramen of Monro)
18 Lateral sulcus
19 Claustrum
20 Insular arteries in the cistern of lateral cerebral fossa (insular cistern)
21 Internal capsule (posterior limb)
22 Insula
23 Thalamus
24 Globus pallidus (pallidum)
25 Pineal gland
26 Putamen
27 Caudate nucleus (tail)
28 Transverse temporal gyrus
29 Internal cerebral vein
30 Hippocampus
31 Vermis of cerebellum
32 Lateral ventricle (trigone with choroid plexus)
33 Straight sinus
34 Middle temporal gyrus
35 Parietal bone
36 Parieto-occipital sulcus
37 Superior sagittal sinus
38 Occipital gyri
39 Occipital bone
40 Striate cortex
41 Occipital pole

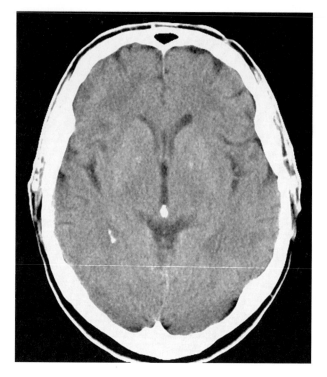

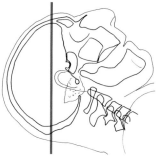

Frontal lobe
Temporal lobe
Occipital lobe
Cerebellum
Mesencephalon

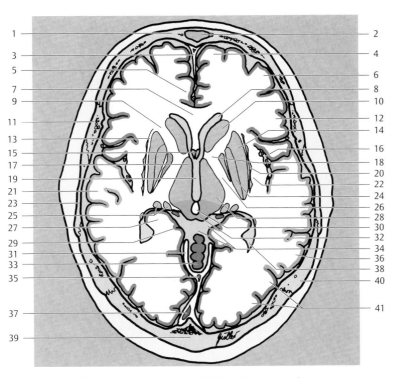

1 Frontal bone
2 Frontal sinus
3 Falx cerebri
4 Superior frontal gyrus
5 Cingulate gyrus
6 Middle frontal gyrus
7 Corpus callosum (genu)
8 Lateral ventricle (anterior horn)
9 Internal capsule (anterior limb)
10 Caudate nucleus (head)
11 Parietal bone
12 Inferior frontal gyrus
13 External capsule
14 Putamen
15 Septum verum
    (precommissural septum)
16 Cistern of lateral cerebral fossa
    (insular cistern)
17 Hypothalamus
18 Internal capsule (genu)
19 Third ventricle
20 Claustrum

21 Superior temporal gyrus
22 Extreme capsule
23 Temporal bone
24 Globus pallidus (pallidum)
25 Geniculate body
26 Internal capsule (posterior limb)
27 Hippocampus
28 Thalamus
29 Parahippocampal gyrus
30 Pineal gland (calcified)
31 Tentorium cerebelli
32 Quadrigeminal plate (colliculus)
33 Vermis of cerebellum
34 Quadrigeminal
    and ambient cisterns
35 Straight sinus
36 Middle temporal gyrus
37 Superior sagittal sinus
38 Lateral ventricle (trigone)
39 Occipital bone
40 Parietal bone
41 Occipital gyri

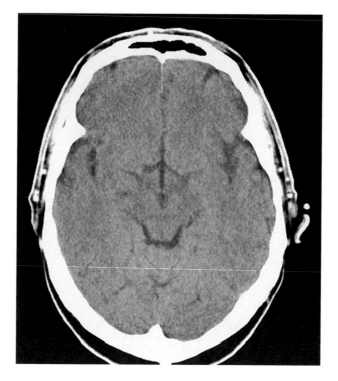

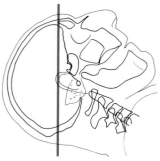

- ◼ Frontal lobe
- ◼ Temporal lobe
- ◼ Occipital lobe
- ◼ Cerebellum
- ◼ Mesencephalon

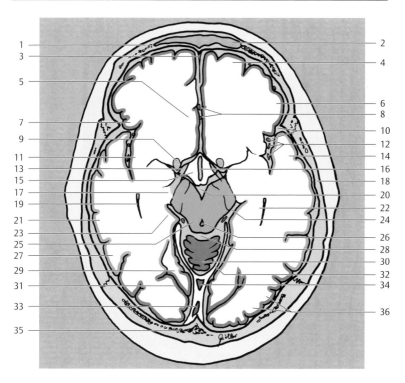

1 Frontal bone
2 Frontal sinus
3 Falx cerebri
4 Superior frontal gyrus
5 Cingulate gyrus
6 Middle frontal gyrus
7 Inferior frontal gyrus
8 Anterior cerebral artery
9 Striatum (inferior portion)
10 Lateral sulcus (insular cistern)
11 Insula
12 Insular arteries
13 Optic tract
14 Superior temporal gyrus
15 Hypothalamus
16 Third ventricle
17 Cerebral peduncle
18 Parietal bone
19 Lateral ventricle
    (temporal horn)
20 Interpeduncular cistern
21 Middle temporal gyrus
22 Hippocampus
23 Parahippocampal gyrus
24 Ambient cistern
25 Mesencephalon (quadrigeminal
    plate)
26 Aqueduct
27 Inferior temporal gyrus
28 Quadrigeminal cistern
29 Lateral occipitotemporal gyrus
30 Vermis of cerebellum
    (superior portion)
31 Parieto-occipital sulcus
32 Tentorium cerebelli
33 Superior sagittal sinus
34 Straight sinus
35 Occipital bone
36 Occipital gyri

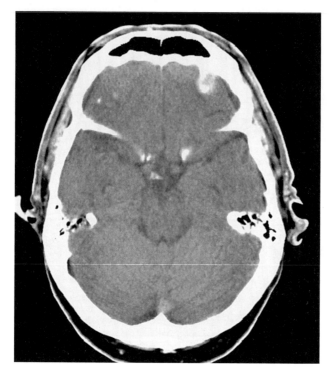

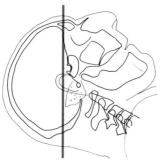

- Frontal lobe
- Temporal lobe
- Cerebellum
- Pons

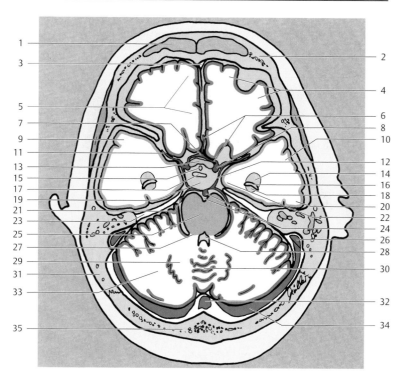

1 Frontal sinus
2 Frontal bone
3 Falx cerebri
4 Orbital gyri
5 Straight gyrus
6 Anterior cerebral artery
7 Anterior communicating artery
8 Internal carotid artery
9 Superior temporal gyrus
10 Middle temporal gyrus
11 Middle cerebral artery
12 Posterior communicating artery
13 Optic chiasm
14 Amygdaloid body
15 Pituitary stalk
16 Lateral ventricle (temporal horn)
17 Dorsum sellae
18 Hippocampus
19 Pentagon of basal cisterns
20 Inferior temporal gyrus
21 Posterior cerebral artery
22 Parahippocampal gyrus
23 Tentorium cerebelli
24 Basilar artery and basal sulcus
25 Pons
26 Sigmoid sinus
27 Cerebellar peduncle (middle)
28 Fourth ventricle
29 Dentate nucleus
30 Vermis of cerebellum (superior part)
31 Temporal bone
32 Confluence of the sinuses
33 Cerebellar hemisphere
34 Transverse sinus
35 Occipital bone

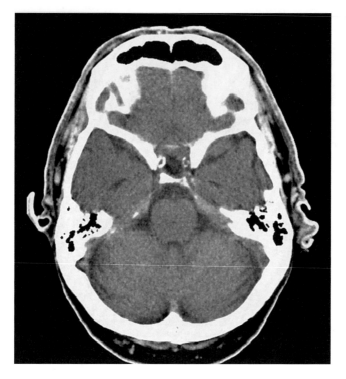

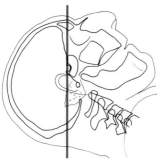

Frontal lobe
Temporal lobe
Cerebellum
Pons

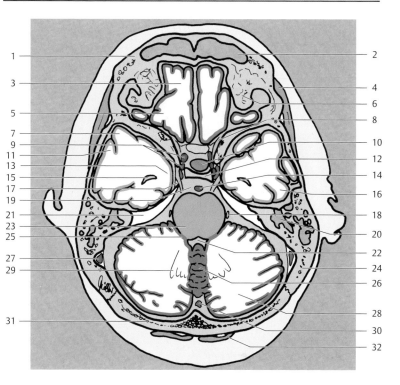

1 Frontal bone
2 Frontal sinus
3 Straight gyrus
4 Temporal muscle
5 Orbital gyri
6 Roof of orbit
7 Superior temporal gyrus
8 Optic nerve
9 Internal carotid artery
10 Pituitary gland
11 Middle temporal gyrus
12 Dorsum sellae
13 Parahippocampal gyrus
14 Basilar artery
15 Lateral ventricle (temporal horn)
16 Inferior temporal gyrus
17 Trigeminal nerve (V)
18 Trochlear nerve
19 Pontine cistern
20 Mastoid antrum
21 Tentorium cerebelli
22 Fourth ventricle
23 Pons
24 Temporal bone
25 Cerebellar peduncle
26 Vermis of cerebellum
27 Sigmoid sinus
28 Cerebellar hemisphere
29 Dentate nucleus
30 Occipital sinus
31 Occipital bone
32 Semispinalis capitis muscle

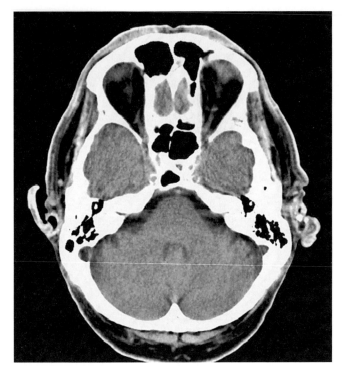

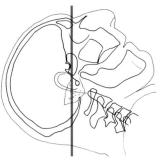

Frontal lobe
Temporal lobe
Cerebellum
Pons

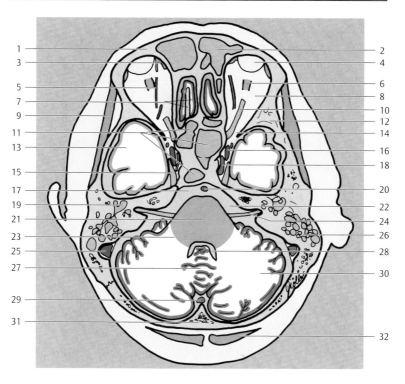

1 Frontal bone
2 Frontal sinus
3 Superior oblique muscle
4 Eyeball
5 Ophthalmic vein
6 Superior rectus muscle
7 Straight gyrus and olfactory bulb
8 Retro-orbital fatty tissue
9 Temporal muscle
10 Optic nerve
11 Sphenoidal sinus
12 Sphenoidal bone
13 Inferior temporal gyrus
14 Superior orbital fissure
15 Trigeminal nerve (ganglion)
16 Internal carotid artery
17 Pontine cistern
18 Cavernous sinus
19 Mastoid antrum
20 Basilar artery
21 Pons
22 Pontocerebellar cistern
23 Middle and inferior cerebellar peduncle
24 Internal auditory meatus with facial (VII) and vestibulocochlear/acoustic (VIII) nerves
25 Sigmoid sinus
26 Mastoid process with mastoid cells
27 Vermis of cerebellum
28 Fourth ventricle
29 Occipital sinus
30 Cerebellar hemisphere
31 Occipital bone
32 Semispinalis capitis muscle

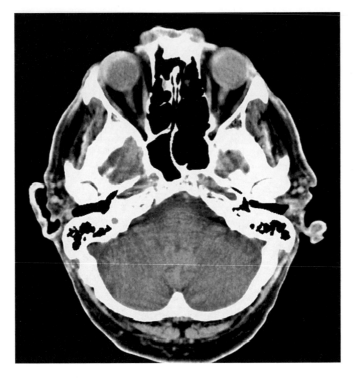

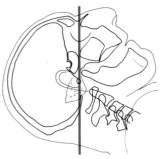

▨	Frontal lobe
▨	Temporal lobe
▨	Cerebellum
▨	Pons

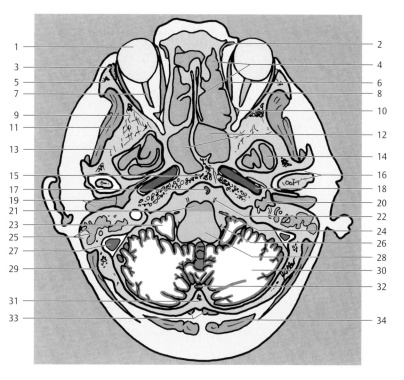

1 Eyeball
2 Superior oblique muscle
3 Lacrimal gland
4 Ethmoidal cells
5 Zygomatic bone
6 Medial rectus muscle
7 Optic nerve
8 Lateral rectus muscle of eyeball
9 Sphenoidal bone
10 Superior rectus muscle
11 Temporal muscle
12 Sphenoidal sinus
13 Temporal bone
14 Temporal lobe (base)
15 Clivus
16 Temporomandibular joint and head of mandible
17 Basilar artery
18 Internal carotid artery
19 External auditory meatus and eardrum (tympanic membrane)
20 Tympanic cavity
21 Pons
22 Abducent nerve (VI)
23 Flocculus
24 Anterior inferior cerebellar artery
25 Mastoid process and mastoid cells
26 Glossopharyngeal (IX) and vagus (X) nerves
27 Sigmoid sinus
28 Medulla oblongata (myelencephalon)
29 Splenius capitis muscle
30 Cerebellar hemisphere
31 Occipital bone
32 Occipital sinus
33 Rectus capitis posterior minor muscle
34 Semispinalis capitis muscle

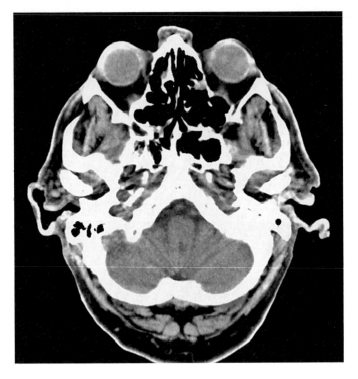

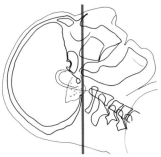

█ Cerebellum
░ Medulla oblongata

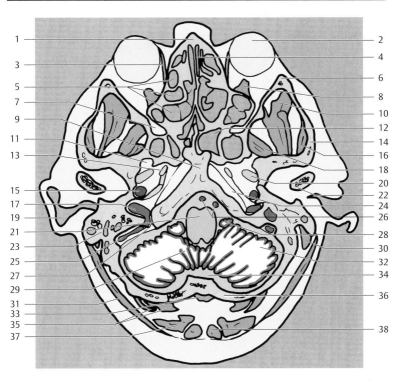

1 Nasal bone
2 Eyeball
3 Medial rectus muscle
4 Nasal septum
5 Ethmoidal cells
6 Zygomatic bone
7 Pterygopalatine fossa
8 Inferior rectus muscle
9 Occipital bone (basilar part)
10 Temporal muscle
11 Foramen ovale with mandibular nerve
12 Sphenoidal sinus
13 Temporal bone (apex of the petrous pyramid)
14 Zygomatic arch
15 Internal carotid artery
16 Masseter muscle
17 Jugular vein (bulb)
18 Lateral pterygoid muscle (superior head)

19 External auditory meatus
20 Auditory tube
21 Medulla oblongata
22 Head of mandible
23 Mastoid process
24 Foramen lacerum
25 Sigmoid sinus
26 Vertebral arteries
27 Petro-occipital fissure
28 Flocculus
29 Cerebellar tonsil
30 Digastric muscle
31 Splenius capitis muscle
32 Cerebellar hemisphere (caudal lobe)
33 Rectus capitis posterior minor muscle
34 Cisterna magna (posterior cerebello-medullary cistern)
35 Rectus capitis posterior major muscle
36 Occipital bone
37 Semispinalis capitis muscle
38 Trapezius muscle

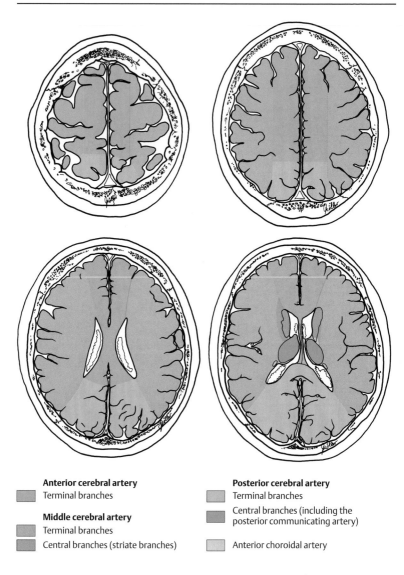

Anterior cerebral artery
Terminal branches

Middle cerebral artery
Terminal branches
Central branches (striate branches)

Posterior cerebral artery
Terminal branches
Central branches (including the posterior communicating artery)

Anterior choroidal artery

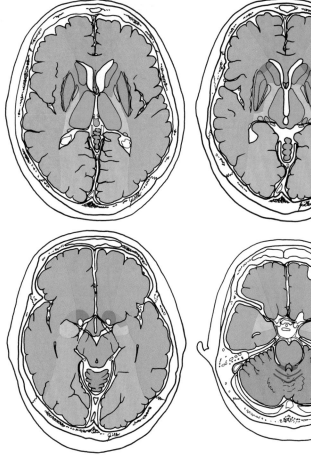

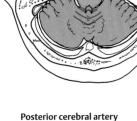

Anterior cerebral artery
Terminal branches

Central branches (striate branches)

Middle cerebral artery
Terminal branches

Central branches (striate branches)

Posterior cerebral artery
Terminal branches

Central branches (including the posterior communicating artery)

Anterior choroidal artery

Superior cerebellar artery

Anterior inferior cerebellar artery

Border region

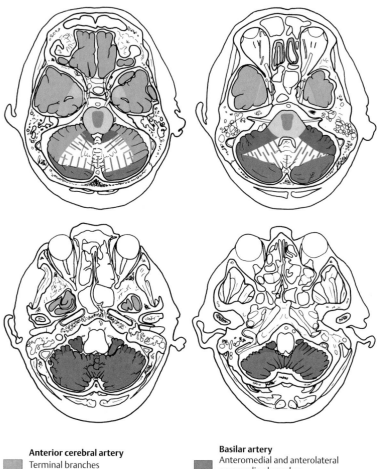

Anterior cerebral artery
Terminal branches

Middle cerebral artery
Terminal branches

Posterior cerebral artery
Terminal branches

Anterior choroidal artery

Basilar artery
Anteromedial and anterolateral
paramedian branches
Circumferential arteries and
Lateral and dorsal paramedian
branches

Superior cerebellar artery

Anterior superior cerebellar artery

Border region

Posterior inferior cerebellar artery

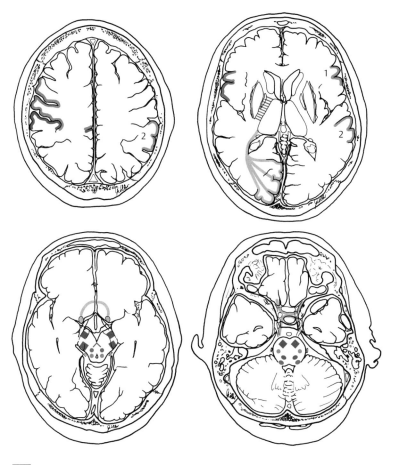

Motor system

Sensory system

Medial lemniscal tract

Spinothalamic tract

Mesencephalic nucleus of
trigeminal nerve

Oculomotor nucleus and
pathways

Optic tract

Speech center
(1 = motor, 2 = sensory)

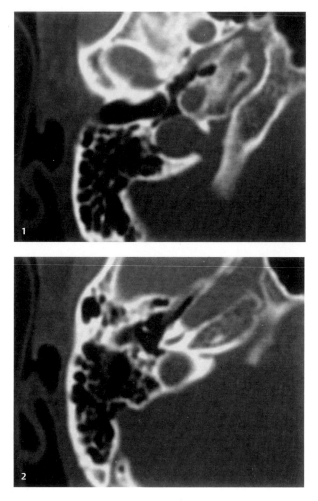

Frontal

Lateral ☐ Medial

Occipital

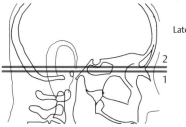

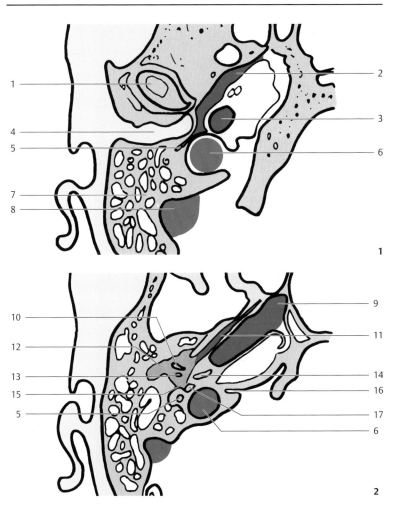

1

2

1 Temporomandibular joint (glenoid roof and articular disc)
2 Pharyngotympanic tube (auditory tube)
3 Internal carotid artery
4 External acoustic meatus
5 Facial canal
6 Internal jugular vein
7 Mastoid process
8 Sigmoid sinus

9 Carotid canal
10 Malleus (handle)
11 Tensor tympani muscle (canal)
12 Middle ear
13 Incus (long limb)
14 Cochlea (basal turn)
15 Sinus tympani
16 Vestibular aqueduct
17 Round window

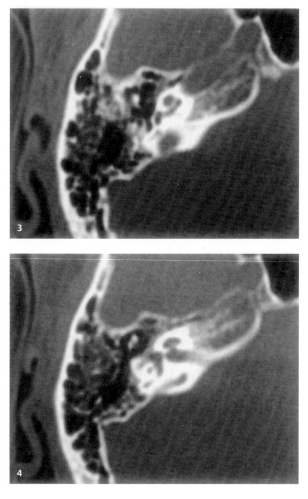

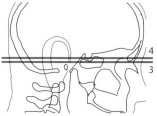

Frontal

Lateral ☐ Medial

Occipital

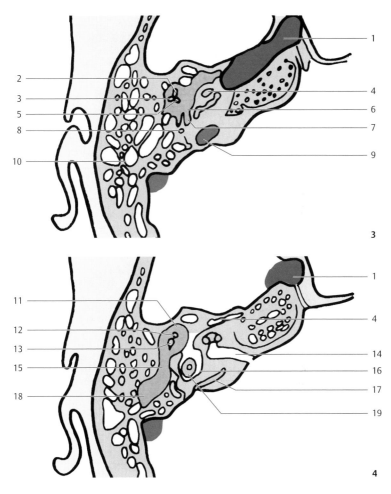

3

4

1 Internal carotid artery (canal)
2 Malleus (handle)
3 Incus (long limb)
4 Cochlea
5 Stapes
6 Oval window
7 Sinus tympani
8 Facial canal
9 Internal jugular vein (bulb)
10 Mastoid

11 Epitympanic recess
12 Malleus (head)
13 Incus (short limb)
14 Internal acoustic meatus
15 Aditus to mastoid antrum
16 Vestibule
17 Posterior semicircular canal
18 Mastoid antrum
19 Lateral semicircular canal

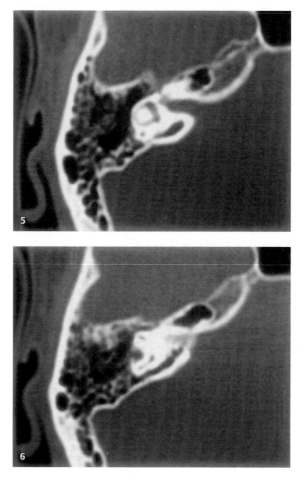

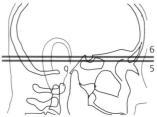

Frontal

Lateral | | Medial

Occipital

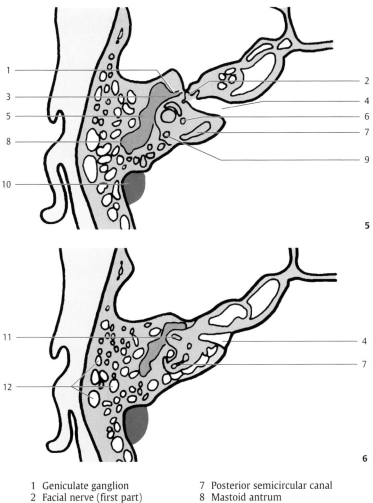

5

6

1 Geniculate ganglion
2 Facial nerve (first part)
3 Facial nerve (second part)
4 Internal acoustic meatus
5 Tympanic cavity
6 Vestibule

7 Posterior semicircular canal
8 Mastoid antrum
9 Lateral semicircular canal
10 Sigmoid sinus
11 Anterior (superior) semicircular canal
12 Mastoid cells

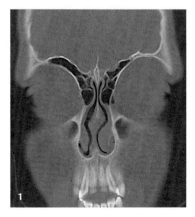

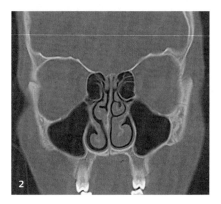

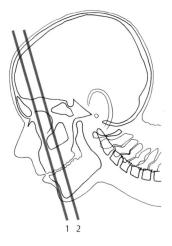

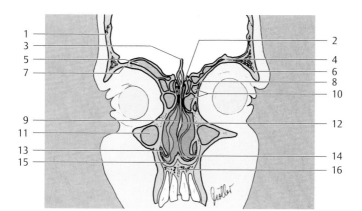

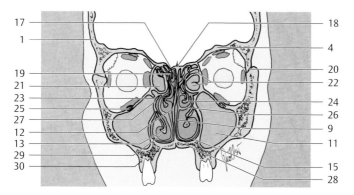

1 Frontal bone	16 Alveolar process of maxilla
2 Cribriform plate	17 Ethmoidal notch
3 Crista galli	18 Ethmoidal bone (cribriform plate)
4 Roof of orbit	19 Superior nasal concha
5 Frontal sinus	20 Frontozygomatic suture
6 Zygomatic process	21 Orbital plate of ethmoidal labyrinth
7 Supraorbital notch	22 Ethmoidal cells (middle)
8 Orbital plate	23 Maxillary hiatus
9 Nasal cavity	24 Middle nasal concha
10 Anterior ethmoidal cells	25 Infraorbital foramen
11 Maxillary sinus	26 Middle nasal meatus
12 Nasal septum	27 Uncinate process
13 Inferior nasal concha	28 Hard palate
14 Vomer	29 Inferior nasal concha
15 Inferior nasal meatus	30 Maxilla (alveolar process)

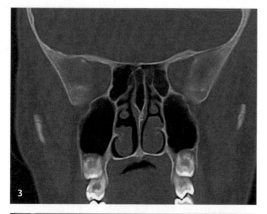

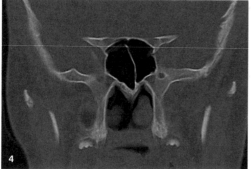

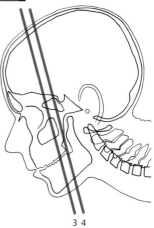

3 4

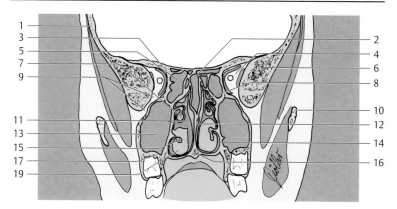

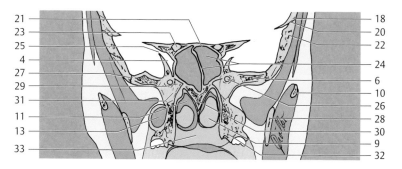

1 Frontal bone
2 Sphenoidal sinus (recess)
3 Sphenoidal bone (lesser wing)
4 Infundibulum of orbit
5 Ethmoidal cells (posterior)
6 Sphenoidal bone (greater wing)
7 Middle nasal concha
8 Superior nasal concha
9 Inferior orbital fissure
10 Zygomatic bone
11 Nasal cavity (common nasal meatus)
12 Nasal septum (perpendicular palate)
13 Maxillary sinus
14 Inferior nasal meatus
15 Inferior nasal concha
16 Palatine bone (horizontal plane)
17 Maxilla (alveolar process)

18 Parietal bone
19 Inferior nasal concha (cavernous body)
20 Squamous suture
21 Sphenoid bone (roof of splenoid sinus)
22 Temporal bone (squamous part)
23 Optic canal
24 Sphenoidal sinus with septum
25 Superior orbital fissure
26 Foramen rotundum of sphenoidal bone
27 Sphenosquamous suture
28 Mandible (body and ramus)
29 Pterygoid canal
30 Ethmoidal bone (nasal septum)
31 Pterygopalatine fossa
32 Pterygoid process
33 Soft palate

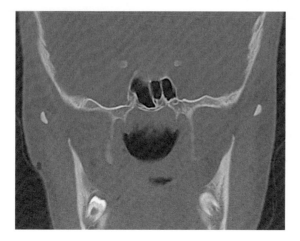

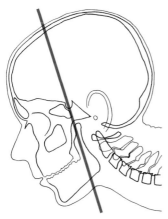

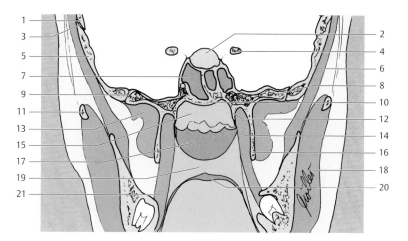

1 Parietal bone
2 Sella turcica
3 Squamous suture
4 Anterior clinoid process
   (sphenoidal bone)
5 Temporal bone (squamous
   part)
6 Temporal muscle
7 Sphenoidal sinus
8 Temporal bone (with articular
   tubercle)
9 Sphenosquamous suture

10 Sphenoidal bone
11 Zygomatic arch
12 Pterygoid process (medial plate)
13 Lateral pterygoid muscle
14 Pterygoid fossa
15 Pharyngeal tonsil
16 Pterygoid process (lateral plate)
17 Nasopharynx
18 Masseter muscle
19 Soft palate
20 Oropharynx (isthmus of fauces)
21 Medial pterygoid muscle

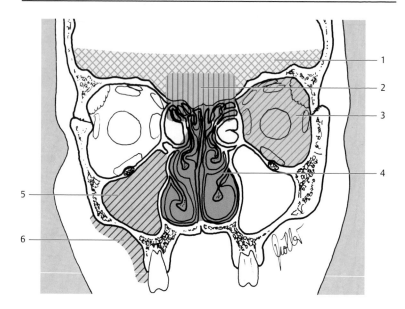

1 Anterior cranial fossa
2 Base of the nose
3 Orbital cavity
4 Nasal cavity
5 Maxillary sinus
6 Buccal space

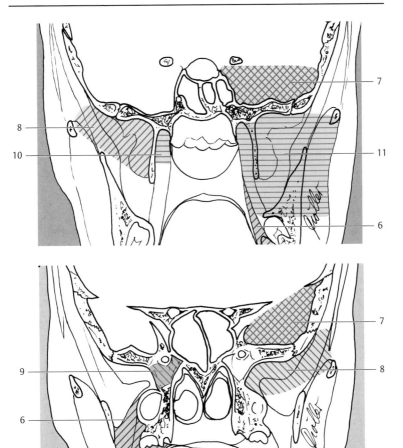

 6 Buccal space
7 Middle cranial fossa
8 Infratemporal fossa
9 Pterygopalatine fossa
10 Pterygoid fossa
11 Masticatory space

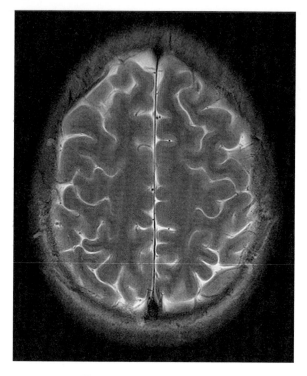

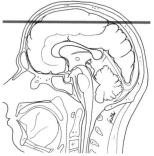

Frontal lobe
Parietal lobe

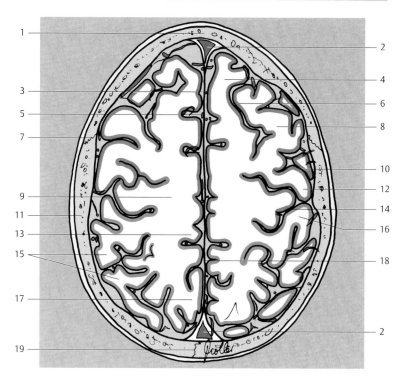

1 Frontal bone
2 Superior sagittal sinus
3 Longitudinal cerebral fissure
4 Superior frontal gyrus
5 Supratrochlear artery (posteromedial)
6 Superior frontal sulcus
7 Coronal suture
8 Middle frontal gyrus
9 Cerebral white matter
   (semioval center)

10 Precentral sulcus
11 Parietal bone
12 Precentral gyrus
13 Paracentral lobule
14 Central sulcus
15 Superior parietal lobule
16 Postcentral gyrus
17 Precuneus
18 Falx cerebri
19 Sagittal suture

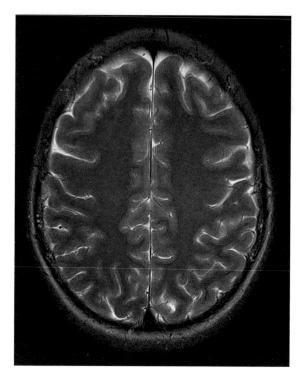

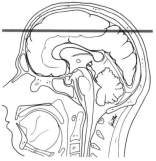

Frontal lobe
Parietal lobe
Occipital lobe

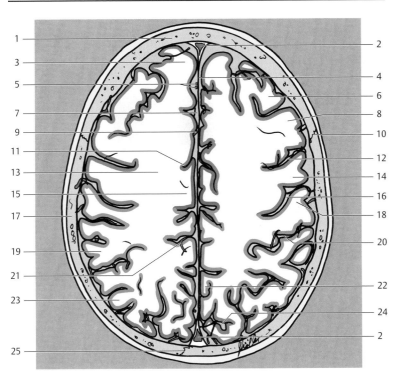

1 Frontal bone
2 Superior sagittal sinus
3 Superior frontal gyrus
4 Falx cerebri
5 Supratrochlear artery
   (mediomedial)
6 Middle frontal gyrus
7 Longitudinal cerebral fissure
8 Inferior frontal gyrus
9 Callosomarginal artery
10 Coronal suture
11 Cingulate sulcus
12 Precentral sulcus
13 Cerebral white matter
   (semioval center)
14 Precentral gyrus
15 Cingulate gyrus and cingulum
16 Central sulcus (fissure of Rolando)
17 Parietal bone
18 Postcentral gyrus
19 Supramarginal gyrus
20 Postcentral sulcus
21 Paracentral branches of
   callosomarginal artery
22 Precuneus
23 Angular gyrus
24 Parieto-occipital sulcus
25 Sagittal suture

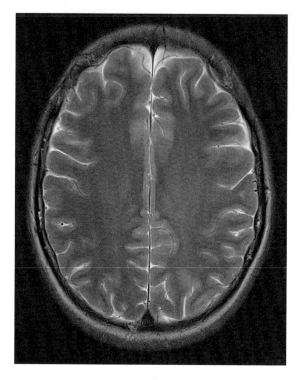

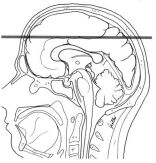

Frontal lobe
Parietal lobe
Occipital lobe

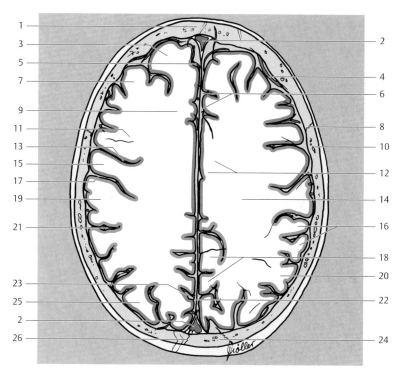

1 Frontal bone
2 Superior sagittal sinus
3 Superior frontal gyrus
4 Superior cerebral vein
5 Supratrochlear (mediomedial) artery
6 Longitudinal cerebral fissure
7 Middle frontal gyrus
8 Coronal suture
9 Callosomarginal artery
10 Parietal bone
11 Inferior frontal gyrus
12 Cingulate gyrus and cingulum
13 Precentral sulcus
14 Cerebral white matter (semioval center)
15 Precentral gyrus
16 Supramarginal gyrus
17 Central sulcus
18 Precuneus
19 Postcentral gyrus
20 Angular gyrus
21 Postcentral sulcus
22 Falx cerebri
23 Parieto-occipital sulcus
24 Occipital bone
25 Occipital gyri
26 Lambdoid suture

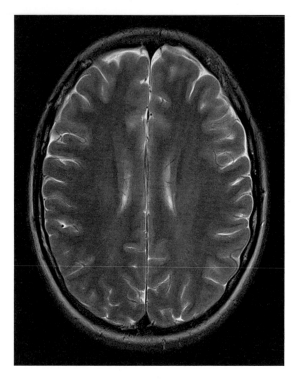

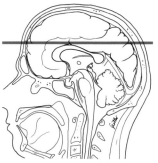

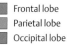

Frontal lobe
Parietal lobe
Occipital lobe

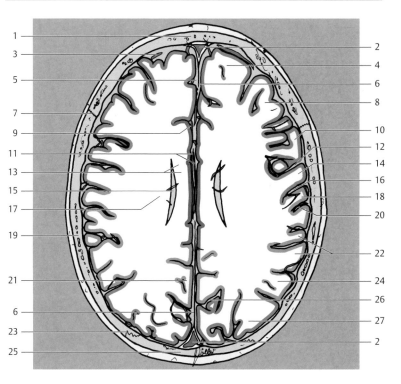

1 Frontal bone	15 Lateral ventricle (central part)
2 Superior sagittal sinus	16 Central sulcus
3 Superior cerebral vein	17 Corona radiata
4 Superior frontal gyrus	18 Postcentral gyrus
5 Longitudinal cerebral fissure	19 Parietal bone
6 Falx cerebri	20 Postcentral sulcus
7 Coronal suture	21 Precuneus
8 Middle frontal gyrus	22 Supramarginal gyrus
9 Callosomarginal artery	23 Lambdoid suture
10 Inferior frontal gyrus	24 Angular gyrus
11 Pericallosal artery	25 Occipital bone
12 Precentral sulcus	26 Parieto-occipital sulcus
13 Cingulate gyrus and cingulum	27 Occipital gyri
14 Precentral gyrus	

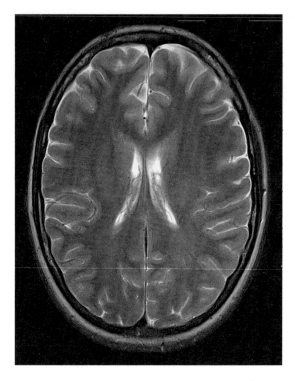

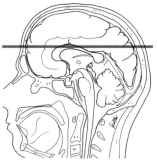

Frontal lobe
Parietal lobe
Occipital lobe

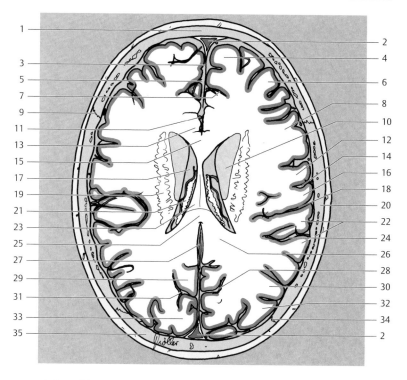

1 Frontal bone
2 Superior sagittal sinus
3 Falx cerebri
4 Superior frontal gyrus
5 Longitudinal cerebral
6 Middle frontal gyrus
7 Cingulate sulcus
8 Inferior frontal gyrus
9 Coronal suture
10 Head of caudate nucleus
11 Pericallosal artery
12 Precentral gyrus
13 Cingulate gyrus
14 Central sulcus
15 Corpus callosum (genu)
16 Postcentral gyrus
17 Lateral ventricle
18 Lateral sulcus
19 Corona radiata
20 Parietal bone
21 Choroid plexus
22 Supramarginal gyrus
23 Fornix
24 Lateral sulcus (posterior ramus)
25 Corpus callosum, splenium
26 Major forceps (occipital forceps)
27 Inferior sagittal sinus
28 Parieto-occipital sulcus
29 Precuneus
30 Angular gyrus
31 Parieto-occipital artery
32 Occipital gyri
33 Cuneus
34 Lambdoid suture
35 Occipital bone

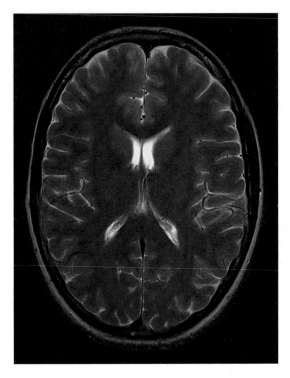

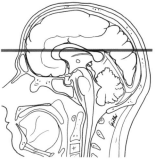

▨	Frontal lobe
▨	Temporal lobe
▨	Parietal lobe
▨	Occipital lobe

1 Frontal bone
2 Superior sagittal sinus
3 Falx cerebri
4 Superior frontal gyrus
5 Cingulate sulcus
6 Cingulate gyrus

7 Pericallosal artery
8 Middle frontal gyrus
9 Corpus callosum (genu)
10 Lateral ventricle (frontal horn)
11 Head of caudate nucleus
12 Inferior frontal gyrus

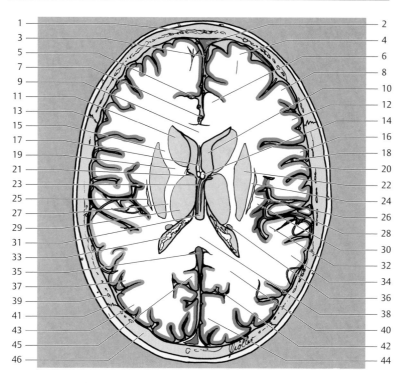

13 Coronal suture
14 Fornix (column)
15 Internal capsule (anterior limb)
16 Precentral gyrus
17 Cave of septum pellucidum
18 Central sulcus
19 Internal capsule (genu)
20 Postcentral gyrus
21 Interventricular foramen
   (foramen of Monro)
22 Putamen
23 Internal cerebral vein
24 External capsule
25 Claustrum
26 Extreme capsule
27 Internal capsule (posterior
   limb)
28 Lateral sulcus
29 Thalamus

30 Insula
31 Third ventricle (suprapineal recess)
32 Transverse temporal gyrus
33 Choroid plexus in trigone of posterior
   horn of lateral ventricle
34 Superior temporal gyrus
35 Great cerebral vein
36 Tail of caudate nucleus
37 Angular gyrus
38 Corpus callosum, splenium
39 Parietal bone
40 Major forceps (occipital forceps)
41 Lambdoid suture
42 Parieto-occipital sulcus
43 Occipital gyri
44 Cuneus
45 Precuneus
46 Occipital bone

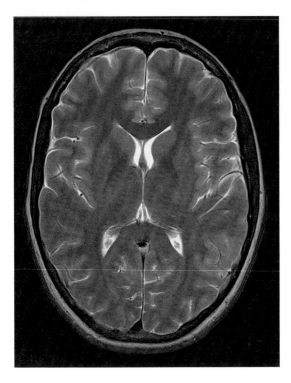

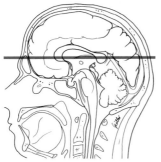

Frontal lobe
Temporal lobe
Parietal lobe
Occipital lobe

1 Frontal bone
2 Superior sagittal sinus
3 Falx cerebri
4 Superior frontal gyrus
5 Cingulate gyrus
6 Middle frontal gyrus
7 Pericallosal artery
8 Coronal suture
9 Corpus callosum (genu)
10 Inferior frontal gyrus

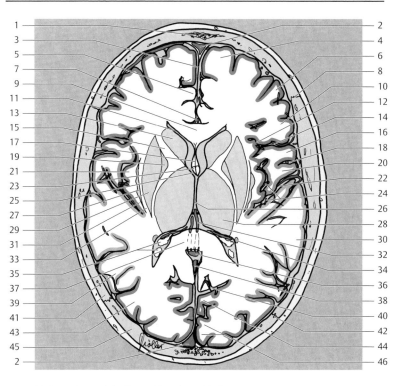

11 Lateral ventricle (frontal horn)
12 Circular sulcus of insula
13 Head of caudate nucleus
14 Lateral sulcus
15 Internal capsule (anterior limb)
16 Precentral gyrus
17 Cave of septum pellucidum
18 Central sulcus
19 Globus pallidus
20 Postcentral gyrus
21 Insula
22 Cistern of lateral cerebral fossa
   (insular cistern)
23 Fornix (column)
24 Insular arteries
25 Interventricular foramen
   (foramen of Monro)
26 Third ventricle
27 Claustrum
28 Thalamus

29 Putamen
30 Superior temporal gyrus
31 Extreme capsule
32 Internal cerebral vein
33 External capsule
34 Tail of caudate nucleus
35 Choroid plexus in trigone of posterior
   horn of lateral ventricle
36 Great cerebral vein
37 Corpus callosum, splenium
38 Straight sinus
39 Middle temporal gyrus
40 Parieto-occipital sulcus
41 Parietal bone
42 Lambdoid suture
43 Occipital gyri
44 Cuneus
45 Occipital bone
46 Striate cortex

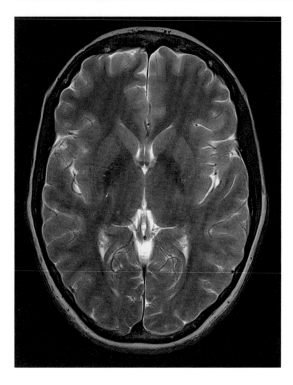

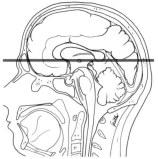

Frontal lobe
Temporal lobe
Parietal lobe
Occipital lobe

1 Frontal bone
2 Superior sagittal sinus
3 Falx cerebri
4 Superior frontal gyrus
5 Cingulate gyrus

6 Middle frontal gyrus
7 Anterior cerebral artery
8 Coronal suture
9 Lateral ventricle
  (frontal horn)

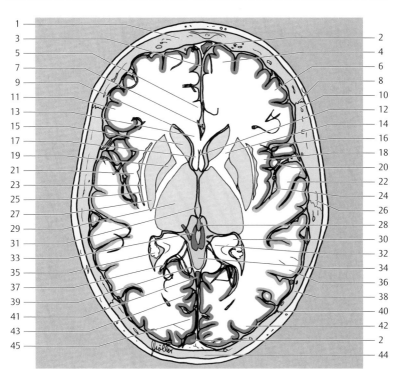

10 Parietal bone
11 Inferior frontal gyrus
12 Cave of septum pellucidum
13 Corpus callosum
14 Internal capsule (anterior limb)
15 Head of caudate nucleus
16 Lateral sulcus
17 Fornix
18 Insula
19 Pallidum
20 Insular arteries
21 Extreme capsule
22 Superior temporal gyrus
23 External capsule
24 Insular cistern
25 Claustrum
26 Temporal bone
27 Putamen
28 Epiphysis of cerebrum

29 Thalamus
30 Hippocampus
31 Third ventricle
32 Uncus of parahippocampal gyrus
33 Internal cerebral vein and
    great cerebral vein
34 Superior cerebellar cistern
35 Choroid plexus in trigone of posterior
    horn of lateral ventricle
36 Middle temporal gyrus
37 Parieto-occipital artery
38 Parietal bone
39 Tentorium cerebelli
40 Lambdoid suture
41 Straight sinus
42 Occipital gyri
43 Cuneus
44 Occipital bone
45 Striate cortex

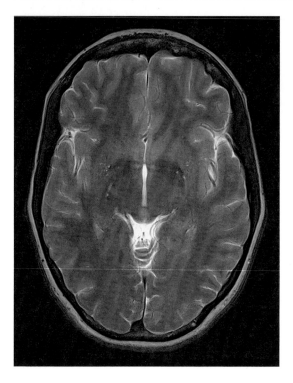

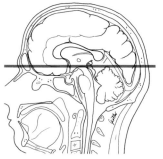

Frontal lobe
Temporal lobe
Occipital lobe
Cerebellum
Mesencephalon

1 Frontal bone
2 Superior frontal gyrus
3 Cingulate gyrus
4 Falx cerebri
5 Anterior cerebral artery

6 Middle frontal gyrus
7 Inferior frontal gyrus
8 Head of caudate nucleus
9 Lateral sulcus
10 Internal capsule (anterior limb)

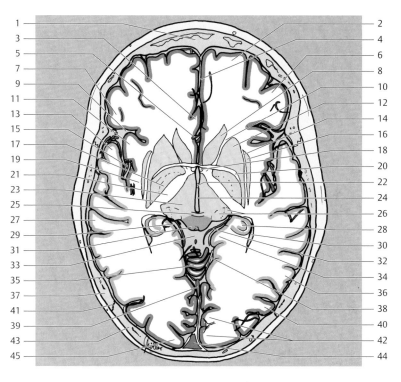

11 Insula
12 Putamen
13 Superior temporal gyrus
14 External capsule
15 Insular arteries
16 Claustrum
17 Globus pallidus (lateral and
    medial segments)
18 Fornix
19 Extreme capsule
20 Anterior commissure
21 Internal capsule (posterior
    limb)
22 Interthalamic adhesion
23 Thalamus
24 Third ventricle
25 Posterior commissure
26 Medial and lateral geniculate
    body

27 Middle temporal gyrus
28 Hippocampus
29 Ambient cistern
30 Lateral ventricle (temporal horn)
31 inferior colliculus
32 Basal vein
33 Quadrigeminal cistern
34 Uncus of parahippocampal gyrus
35 Vermis of superior cerebellar lobe
36 Inferior temporal gyrus
37 Temporal bone
38 Tentorium cerebelli
39 Straight sinus
40 Occipital gyri
41 Lambdoid suture
42 Striate cortex
43 Occipital bone
44 Superior sagittal sinus
45 Occipital pole

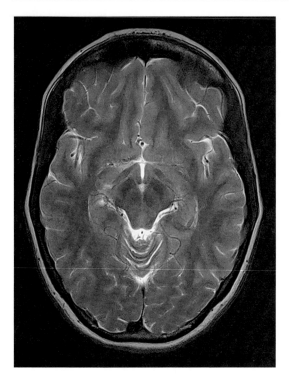

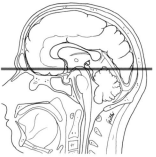

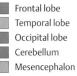

Frontal lobe
Temporal lobe
Occipital lobe
Cerebellum
Mesencephalon

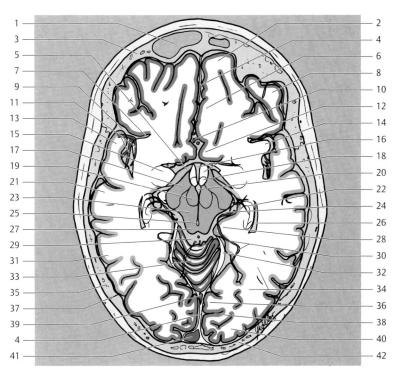

1 Frontal sinus
2 Superior frontal gyrus
3 Frontal bone
4 Falx cerebri
5 Optic tract
6 Cingulate gyrus
7 Circular sulcus of insula
8 Middle frontal gyrus
9 Lateral sulcus
10 Anterior cerebral artery
11 Insular arteries
12 Subcallosal cortex
13 Superior temporal gyrus
14 Insula
15 Amygdaloid body
16 Third ventricle
   (optic recess)
   and hypothalamus
17 Cerebral peduncle
18 Mammillary body
19 Red nucleus
20 Interpeduncular fossa

21 Middle temporal gyrus
22 Hippocampus
23 Tegmentum of midbrain
24 Ambient cistern
25 Aqueduct of mesencephalon
26 Lateral ventricle (temporal horn)
27 Inferior colliculus
28 Uncus of parahippocampal gyrus
29 Quadrigeminal cistern
30 Posterior cerebral artery
31 Inferior temporal gyrus
32 Tentorium cerebelli
33 Anterior cerebellar lobule (Vermis)
34 Optic radiation
35 Temporal bone
36 Striate cortex
37 Lambdoid suture
38 Calcarine sulcus
39 Straight sinus
40 Occipital pole
41 Superior sagittal sinus
42 Occipital bone

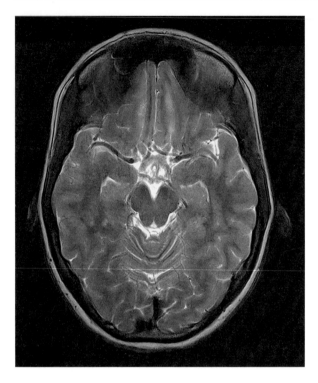

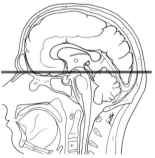

Frontal lobe
Temporal lobe
Cerebellum
Mesencephalon

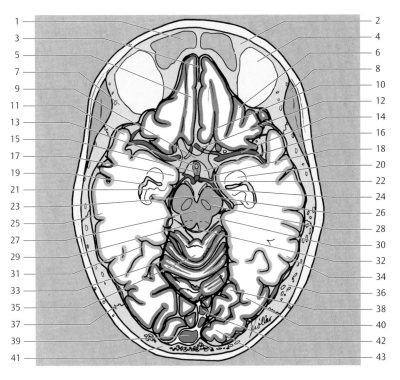

1 Frontal sinus	21 Hippocampus
2 Frontal bone	22 Posterior cerebral artery
3 Falx cerebri	23 Interpeduncular cistern
4 Orbital roof	24 Oculomotor nerve (III)
5 Straight gyrus	25 Middle temporal gyrus
6 Orbital gyrus	26 Cerebral peduncle
7 Sphenoidal bone	27 Tegmentum of midbrain
8 Temporal muscle	28 Substantia nigra
9 Optic chiasm	29 Inferior colliculus
10 Olfactory sulcus	30 Ambient cistern
11 Superior temporal gyrus	31 Collateral sulcus
12 Anterior cerebral artery	32 Aqueduct of midbrain
13 Infundibular recess	33 Tentorium cerebelli
14 Middle cerebral artery	34 Inferior temporal gyrus
15 Hypothalamus	35 Anterior cerebellar lobulus
16 Chiasmatic cistern	36 Temporal bone
17 Uncus of parahippocampal gyrus	37 Lambdoid suture
18 Posterior communicating artery	38 Medial occipitotemporal gyrus
19 Lateral ventricle (temporal horn)	39 Superior sagittal sinus
20 Amygdaloid body	40 Lateral occipitotemporal gyrus
	41 Occipital bone
	42 Straight sinus
	43 Occipital gyri

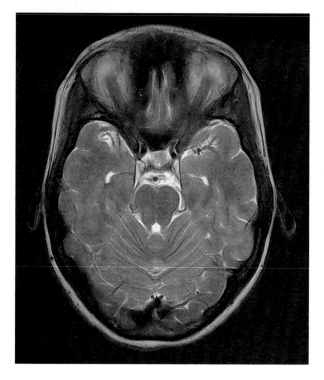

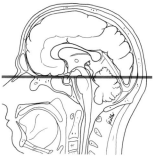

Temporal lobe
Occipital lobe
Cerebellum
Mesencephalon
Pons

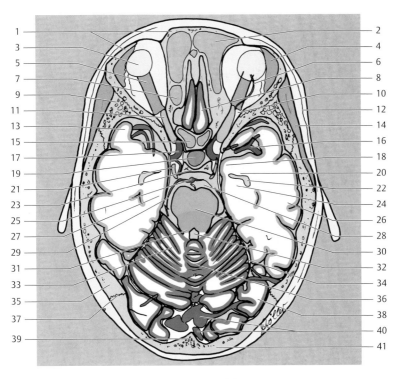

1 Frontal bone	21 Abducent nerve
2 Frontal sinus	22 Lateral ventricle (temporal horn)
3 Eyeball	23 Dorsum sellae
4 Lacrimal gland	24 Hippocampus
5 Superior rectus muscle	25 Basilar artery
6 Ophthalmic vein	26 Middle temporal gyrus
7 Ethmoidal cells	27 Parahippocampal gyrus
8 Straight gyrus	28 Prepontine cistern
9 Sphenoidal bone	29 Posterior cerebral artery
10 Superior orbital fissure	30 Pons
11 Optic nerve	31 Superior cerebellar peduncle
12 Temporoparietal muscle	32 Fourth ventricle
13 Superior temporal gyrus	33 Anterior lobe of cerebellum
14 Temporal muscle	34 Tentorium cerebelli
15 Sphenoidal sinus	35 Temporal bone
16 Middle cerebral artery	36 Vermis of cerebellum
17 Internal carotid artery	37 Lambdoid suture
18 Uncus of parahippocampal gyrus	38 Occipital gyri
19 Pituitary gland	39 Internal occipital protuberance
20 Amygdaloid body	40 Confluence of sinuses
	41 Occipital bone

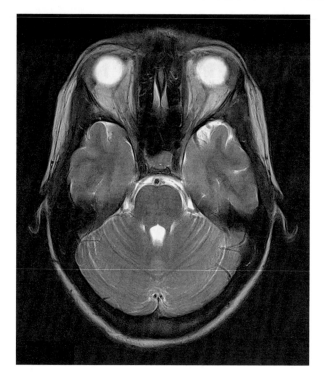

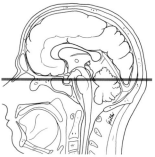

Temporal lobe
Occipital lobe
Cerebellum
Pons

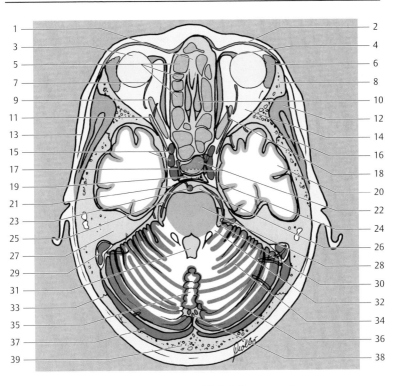

1 Ethmoidal bone
2 Orbicularis oris muscle and occipitofrontal muscle
3 Eyeball
4 Medial rectus muscle
5 Ethmoidal cells
6 Lacrimal gland
7 Superior ophthalmic vein
8 Zygomatic bone
9 Optic nerve
10 Olfactory bulb
11 Oculomotor (III) and abducent (VI) nerves
12 Temporal muscle
13 Temporoparietal muscle
14 Retro-orbital fatty tissue
15 Internal carotid artery
16 Sphenoidal bone
17 Cavernous sinus
18 Ophthalmic artery
19 Dorsum sellae

20 Inferior temporal gyrus
21 Posterior petroclinoid ligament
22 Pituitary gland (neurohypophysis and adenohypophysis)
23 Basilar artery
24 Anterior petroclinoid ligament
25 Posterior cerebral artery
26 Prepontine cistern
27 Petrous part of temporal bone
28 Pons
29 Sigmoid sinus
30 Trigeminal nerve (V)
31 Fourth ventricle
32 Middle cerebellar peduncle
33 Lambdoid suture
34 Anterior lobe of cerebellum
35 Vermis of cerebellum
36 Posterior lobe of cerebellum
37 Transverse sinus
38 Occipital sinus
39 Occipital bone

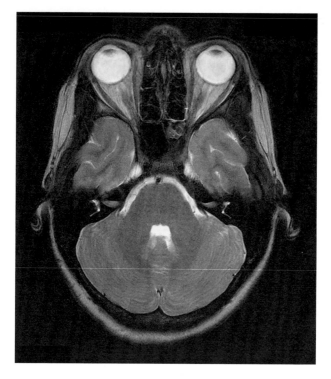

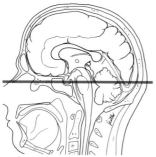

Temporal lobe
Cerebellum
Pons

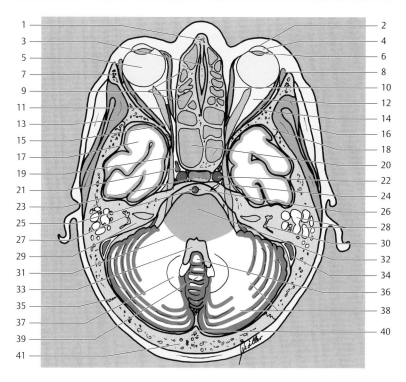

1 Nasal bone	22 Internal carotid artery
2 Cornea	23 Pituitary gland
3 Nasal septum	24 Trigeminal ganglion
4 Anterior chamber of eyeball	25 Basilar artery
5 Eyeball	26 Prepontine cistern
6 Lens	27 Cochlea
7 Zygomatic bone	28 Mastoid cells
8 Lacrimal gland	29 Petrous part of temporal bone
9 Ethmoidal cells	30 Semicircular canal
10 Medial rectus muscle	31 Middle cerebellar peduncle
11 Optic nerve	32 Pons
12 Retro-orbital fatty tissue	33 Fourth ventricle
13 Temporal muscle	34 Sigmoid sinus
14 Lateral rectus muscle	35 Lambdoid suture
15 Ophthalmic artery	36 Uvula of vermis
16 Temporoparietal muscle	37 Dentate nucleus
17 Temporal lobe (temporal pole)	38 Posterior lobe of cerebellum
18 Sphenoidal bone	39 Vermis of cerebellum
19 Oculomotor nerve	40 Internal occipital protuberance
20 Sphenoidal sinus	41 Occipital bone
21 Cavernous sinus	

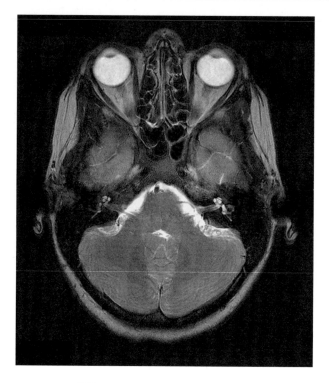

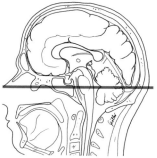

Temporal lobe
Cerebellum
Pons

1 Nasal bone
2 Cornea
3 Ethmoidal cells
4 Anterior chamber of eyeball
5 Eyeball

6 Lens
7 Zygomatic bone
8 Medial rectus muscle
9 Optic nerve
10 Lateral rectus muscle

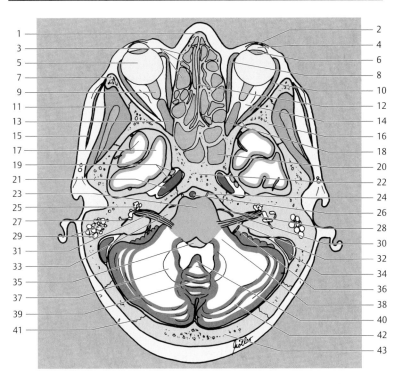

11 Temporal muscle
12 Nasal septum
13 Superior rectus muscle and levator palpebrae superioris muscle
14 Retro-orbital fatty tissue
15 Temporoparietal muscle
16 Sphenoidal bone
17 Temporal pole
18 Superior orbital fissure
19 Maxillary and mandibular nerves
20 Sphenoidal sinus
21 Internal carotid artery
22 Clivus
23 Pons
24 Abducent nerve (VI)
25 Cochlea
26 Basilar artery

27 Posterior semicircular canal
28 Superior cerebellar artery
29 Mastoid cells
30 Facial nerve (VII) and intermediate nerve
31 Internal acoustic meatus
32 Vestibulocochlear (auditory) nerve (VIII)
33 Pontocerebellar cistern
34 Sigmoid sinus
35 Fourth ventricle
36 Anterior inferior cerebellar artery
37 Dentate nucleus
38 Middle cerebellar peduncle
39 Vermis of cerebellum
40 Uvula of vermis
41 Lambdoid suture
42 Caudal lobule of cerebellum
43 Occipital bone

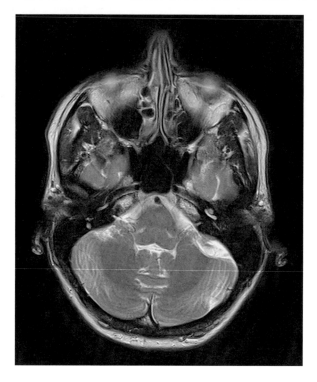

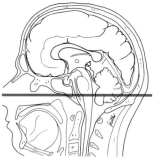

Cerebellum
Pons
Medulla oblongata

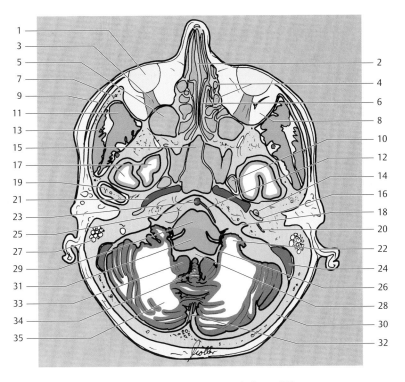

1 Eyeball
2 Nasal septum
3 Inferior rectus muscle
4 Ethmoidal cells
5 Maxillary sinus
6 Nasal sinus
7 Zygomatic bone
8 Retrobulbar fat
9 Orbicularis oris muscle
10 Trigeminal nerve (V)
11 Temporal muscle
12 Anterior inferior cerebellar
    artery
13 Masseter muscle
14 Cochlea
15 Sphenoidal sinus
16 Vestibule
17 Inferior temporal gyrus
18 Internal acoustic meatus

19 Head of mandible
20 Posterior semicircular canal
21 Internal carotid artery
22 Flocculus
23 Basilar artery
24 Transverse sinus
25 Pontocerebellar cistern
26 Lateral aperture of fourth ventricle
    (foramen of Luschka)
27 Mastoid cells
28 Fourth ventricle
29 Pons
30 Occipital bone
31 Medulla oblongata
32 Falx cerebelli
33 Tonsil of cerebellum
34 Vermis of cerebellum
35 Cerebellum

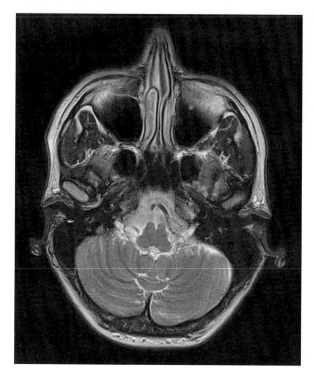

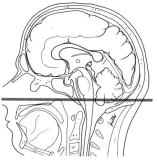

Cerebellum
Medulla oblongata

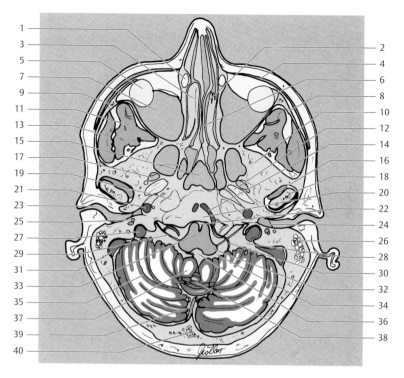

1 Nasolacrimal duct
2 Nasal cavity
3 Nasal concha
4 Orbicularis oris muscle
5 Eyeball
6 Nasal septum
7 Maxillary sinus
8 Sphenoidal bone
9 Zygomatic bone
10 Temporal bone
11 Temporal muscle
12 Pharyngotympanic tube (auditory tube)
13 Masseter muscle
14 Vertebral artery
15 Sphenoidal bone
16 Articular disc
17 Trigeminal nerve (V)
18 Head of mandible
19 Foramen lacerum
20 Clivus
21 Internal carotid artery
22 Ventral median fissure
23 External acoustic meatus
24 Tympanic membrane
25 Cochlea
26 Mastoid cells
27 Internal jugular vein
28 Pontocerebellar cistern
29 Glossopharyngeal nerve (IX) and vagus nerve (X)
30 Anterior inferior cerebellar artery
31 Sigmoid sinus
32 Medulla oblongata (caudal cerebellar peduncle)
33 Medulla oblongata (olivary nucleus)
34 Lateral aperture of fourth ventricle (foramen of Luschka)
35 Cerebellum (posterior lobe)
36 Fourth ventricle
37 Tonsil of cerebellum
38 Vermis of cerebellum
39 Falx cerebelli
40 Occipital bone

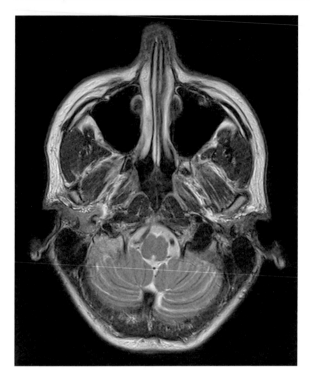

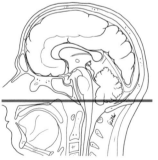

■ Cerebellum
□ Medulla oblongata

1 Nasal bone
2 Nasal septum
3 Superior nasal concha
4 Maxilla (with infra-orbital canal)
5 Levator labii superioris muscle
6 Medial wall of maxillary sinus (with maxillary hiatus)
7 Orbicularis oris muscle
8 Vomer (sphenoidal bone)

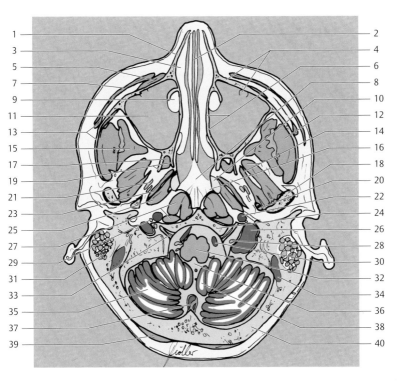

9 Nasolacrimal duct
10 Pharyngotympanic tube (auditory tube)
11 Maxillary sinus
12 Masseter muscle
13 Zygomatic bone and zygomatic muscles
14 Lateral pterygoid muscle (superior and inferior heads)
15 Temporal muscles
16 Pharyngeal recess
17 Medial pterygoid muscle
18 Head of mandible
19 Pterygoid process (medial and lateral plates)
20 Sphenoidal bone (tip)
21 Mandibular nerve and auriculotemporal nerve
22 Internal carotid artery

23 Tensor veli palatini muscle
24 Clivus
25 Levator veli palatini muscle
26 Internal jugular vein (bulb)
27 Longus capitis muscle
28 Vagus (X) and accessory (XI) nerves
29 Glossopharyngeal nerve (IX)
30 Vertebral artery
31 Mastoid cells
32 Medulla oblongata
33 Hypoglossal nerve (XII)
34 Sigmoid sinus
35 Hemisphere of cerebellum (posterior lobe)
36 Fourth ventricle (medial aperture)
37 Falx cerebelli with occipital sinus
38 Tonsil of cerebellum
39 Semispinalis capitis muscle
40 Occipital bone

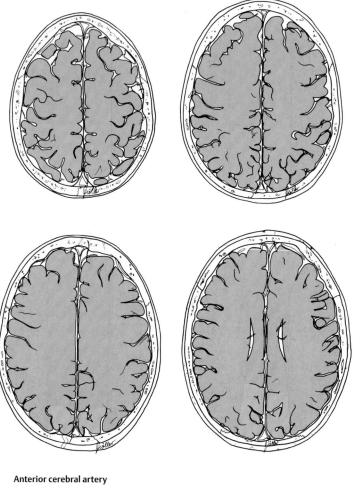

Anterior cerebral artery
Terminal branches

Middle cerebral artery
Terminal branches

Posterior cerebral artery
Terminal branches

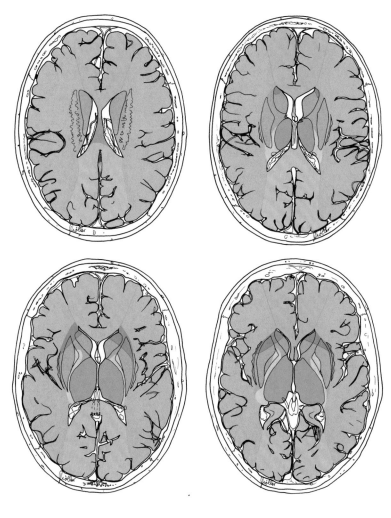

Anterior cerebral artery

Terminal branches

Central branches (striated branches arteries and Huebner's recurrent including distal medial striate artery)

Middle cerebral artery

Terminal branches

Central branches (striated branches)

Posterior cerebral artery

Terminal branches

Central branches (including the posterior communicating artery)

Anterior choroidal artery

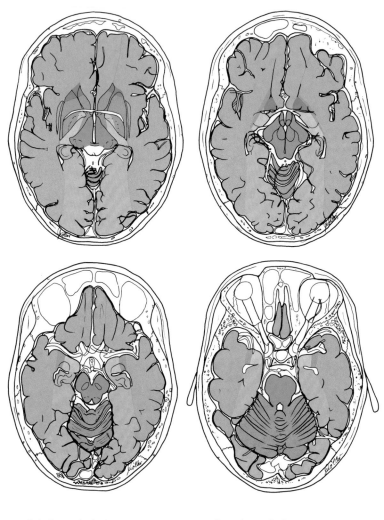

Anterior cerebral artery
Terminal branches

Central branches (striated branches)

Middle cerebral artery
Terminal branches

Central branches (striated branches)

Posterior cerebral artery
Terminal branches

Central branches (including the posterior communicating artery)

Anterior choroidal artery

Superior cerebellar artery

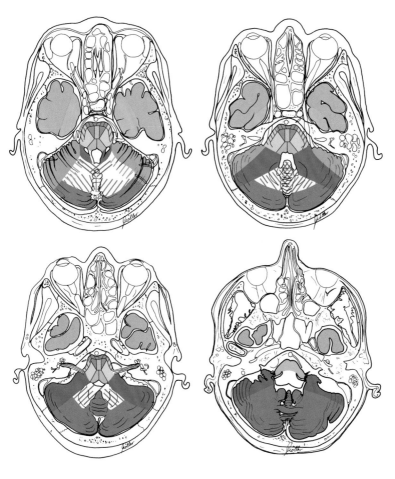

Middle cerebral artery
Terminal branches

Posterior cerebral artery
Terminal branches

Basilar artery: superficial arteries
Median brain-stem arteries
Short circumferential artery
Long circumferential artery

Basilar artery: central arteries
Anteromedial
Anterolateral
Lateral
Dorsal

Superior cerebellar artery
Anterior inferior cerebellar artery
Border region
Posterior inferior cerebellar artery

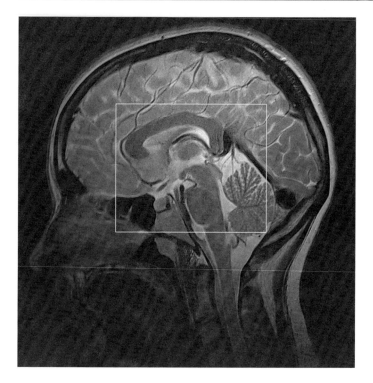

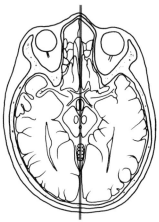

- Frontal lobe
- Parietal lobe
- Occipital lobe
- Cerebellum
- Mesencephalon
- Pons
- Medulla oblongata

1 Superior frontal gyrus
2 Parietal bone and coronal suture
3 Frontal bone
4 Superior sagittal sinus
5 Cingulate gyrus and sulcus
6 Precentral gyrus
7 Corpus callosum (genu)

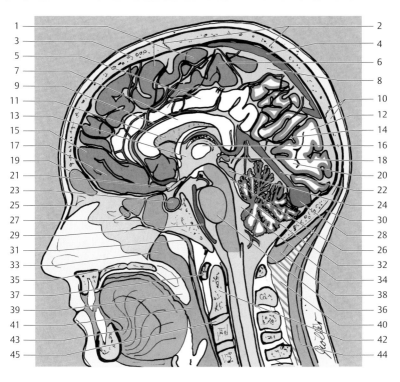

8 Falx cerebri in Longitudinal
   cerebral fissure
9 Pericallosal artery
10 Occipital bone and lambdoid
   suture
11 Septum pellucidum
12 Cuneus
13 Third ventricle
14 Parieto-occipital sulcus
15 Frontal pole
16 Interthalamic adhesion
17 Straight gyrus
18 Cerebral epiphysis
19 Frontal sinus
20 Lingual gyrus
21 Optic nerve (II)
22 Straight sinus
23 Pituitary gland
24 Quadrigeminal plate
25 Nasal bone
26 Aqueduct

27 Ethmoid sinus and sphenoidal sinus
28 Confluence of sinuses
29 Basilar artery
30 External occipital protuberance
31 Superior constrictor muscle of
   pharynx
32 Cerebellum
33 Nasopharynx
34 Fourth ventricle
35 Hard palate
36 Pons
37 Atlas, anterior arch
38 Rectus capitis posterior minor muscle
39 Uvula
40 Ligamentum nuchae (nuchal
   ligament)
41 Oropharynx
42 Dens of axis
43 Tongue
44 Semispinalis capitis muscle
45 Intervertebral disc (C2/C3)

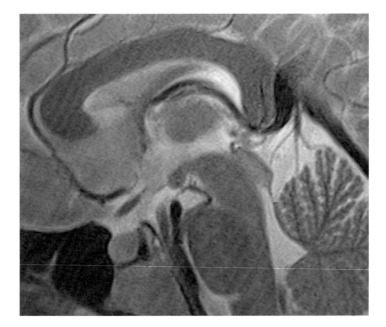

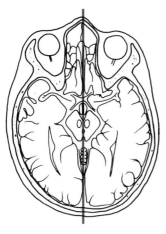

Frontal lobe
Parietal lobe
Occipital lobe
Cerebellum
Mesencephalon
Pons
Medulla oblongata

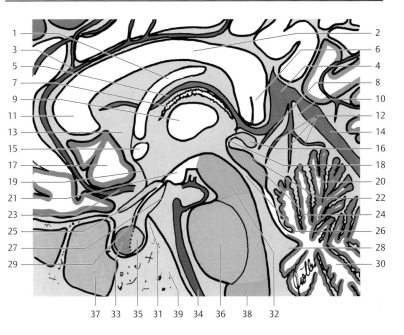

1 Fornix (body)
2 Corpus callosum (trunk)
3 Pericallosal artery
4 Great cerebral vein
5 Internal cerebral vein
6 Corpus callosum (splenium)
7 Choroid plexus
8 Basal vein
9 Interthalamic adhesion
10 Cistern of great cerebral vein
11 Corpus callosum (genu)
12 Cerebellar veins
13 Third ventricle
14 Straight sinus
15 Anterior commissure
16 Pineal body
17 Paraterminal gyrus
18 Posterior commissure
19 Lamina terminalis
20 Hemisphere of cerebellum (anterior lobe)
21 Mammillary body
22 Tectal (quadrigeminal) plate (superior colliculus)
23 Anterior cerebral artery
24 Tectal (quadrigeminal) plate (posterior colliculus)
25 Optic nerve (II)
26 Aqueduct
27 Liliequist's membrane
28 Fourth ventricle (roof)
29 Infundibulum of pituitary gland
30 Hemisphere of cerebellum (posterior lobe)
31 Dorsum sellae
32 Mesencephalon (midbrain)
33 Anterior lobe of pituitary gland (adenohypophysis)
34 Basilar artery
35 Posterior lobe of pituitary gland (neurohypophysis)
36 Pons
37 Sphenoidal sinus
38 Medulla oblongata
39 Clivus

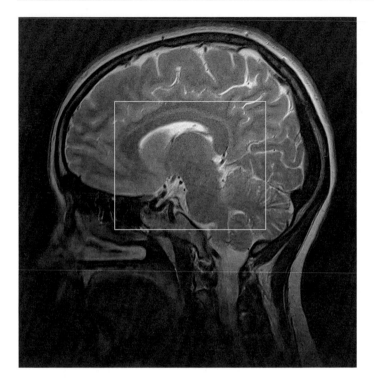

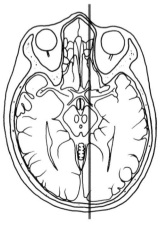

Frontal lobe
Parietal lobe
Occipital lobe
Cerebellum
Mesencephalon
Pons
Medulla oblongata

1 Frontal bone and coronal suture
2 Parietal bone
3 Superior frontal gyrus
4 Precentral gyrus
5 Cingulate gyrus
6 Central sulcus
7 Corpus callosum
8 Postcentral gyrus

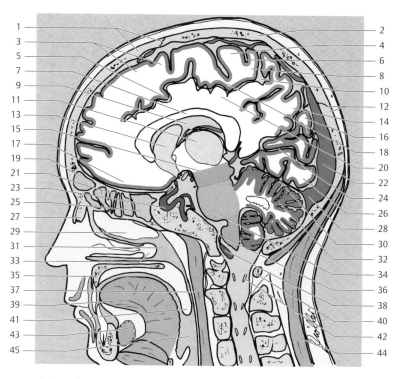

 9 Lateral ventricle (central part)
10 Postcentral sulcus
11 Thalamus
12 Occipital bone and lambdoid
    suture
13 Caudate nucleus (head)
14 Precuneus
15 Cerebral peduncle
16 Cuneus
17 Straight gyrus
18 Precentral lobule
19 Frontal sinus
20 Cingulate gyrus
21 Ethmoidal sinus
22 Superior sagittal sinus
23 Internal carotid artery (syphon)
24 Calcarine sulcus
25 Sphenoidal sinus
26 Medial occipitotemporal gyrus

27 Nasal bone
28 Confluence of sinuses
29 Middle nasal concha
30 Tentorium cerebelli
31 Nasopharynx
32 Cerebellum
33 Inferior nasal concha
34 Pons
35 Hard palate
36 Clivus
37 Longus capitis muscle
38 Vertebral artery
39 Tongue
40 Atlas, posterior arch
41 Uvula
42 Nerve roots
43 Sublingual gland
44 Semispinalis capitis muscle
45 Oropharynx

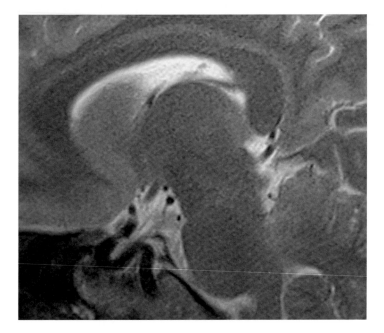

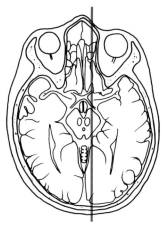

Frontal lobe
Parietal lobe
Occipital lobe
Cerebellum
Mesencephalon
Pons
Medulla oblongata

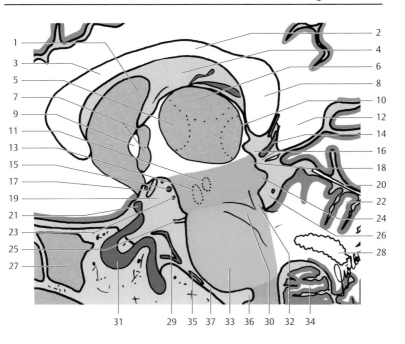

1 Head of caudate nucleus
2 Corpus callosum (trunk)
3 Corpus callosum (genu)
4 Lateral ventricle
5 Thalamus (ventral lateral complex)
6 Thalamus (posterior lateral complex)
7 Globus pallidus (lateral and medial segments)
8 Corpus callosum (splenium)
9 Anterior commissure
10 Thalamus (pulvinar)
11 Red nucleus
12 Parahippocampal gyrus
13 Substantia nigra
14 Great cerebral vein
15 Posterior cerebral artery
16 Quadrigeminal cistern
17 Optic tract
18 Tectal (quadrigeminal) plate (superior colliculus)
19 Interpeduncular cistern
20 Tentorium cerebelli
21 Anterior cerebral artery
22 Hemisphere of cerebellum (anterior lobe)
23 Superior cerebellar artery
24 Tectal (quadrigeminal) plate (posterior colliculus)
25 Trigeminal nerve (V)
26 Ambient cistern
27 Sphenoidal sinus
28 Dentate nucleus
29 Posterior communicating artery
30 Cerebellar peduncle
31 Internal carotid artery
32 Lateral lemniscus
33 Pons
34 Tonsil of cerebellum
35 Abducent nerve (VI)
36 Fourth ventricle (lateral aperture)
37 Pontocerebellar cistern

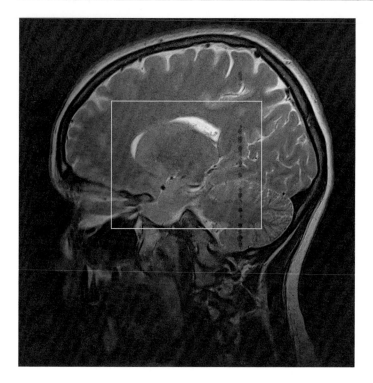

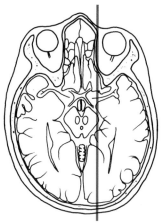

Frontal lobe
Temporal lobe
Parietal lobe
Occipital lobe
Cerebellum
Pons

1 bone
2 Frontal bone and coronal suture
3 Parietal Superior frontal gyrus
4 Precentral gyrus
5 Corpus callosum
6 Postcentral gyrus
7 Caudate nucleus (body)
8 Central sulcus

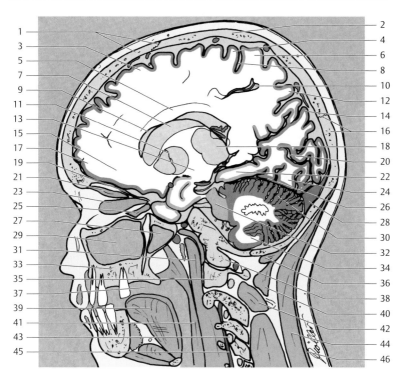

9 Lateral ventricle (frontal horn)
10 Postcentral sulcus
11 Basal nuclei
12 Precuneus
13 Cerebral peduncle
14 Cuneus
15 Orbital gyrus
16 Occipital bone and lambdoid suture
17 Inferior frontal gyrus
18 Thalamus
19 Roof of orbit
20 Calcarine sulcus
21 Superior rectus muscle
22 Parahippocampal gyrus
23 Medial rectus muscle
24 Medial occipitotemporal gyrus
25 Inferior rectus muscle
26 Tentorium cerebelli
27 Sphenoidal sinus

28 Transverse sinus
29 Maxillary sinus
30 Superior cerebellar lobe
31 Longus capitis muscle
32 Middle cerebral peduncle
33 Maxilla
34 Inferior cerebellar lobe
35 Atlas, lateral mass
36 Rectus capitis posterior minor muscle
37 Oropharynx
38 Occipital condyle
39 Tongue
40 Rectus capitis posterior major muscle
41 Middle constrictor muscle of pharynx
42 Obliquus capitis inferior muscle
43 Spinal nerve root C4
44 Splenius capitis muscle
45 Vertebral artery
46 Trapezius muscle

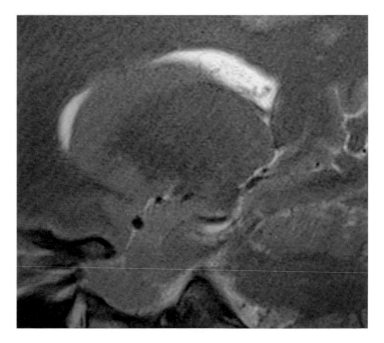

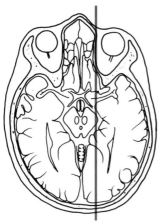

Frontal lobe
Temporal lobe
Parietal lobe
Occipital lobe
Cerebellum
Pons

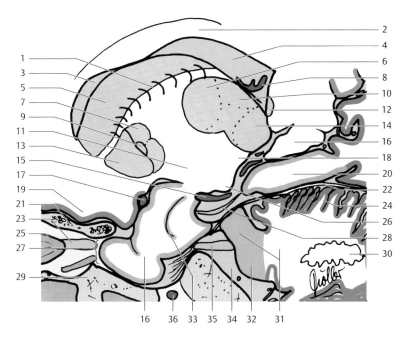

16   36   33   35   34   32   31

1 Corpus striatum
2 Corpus callosum (trunk)
3 Lateral ventricle (frontal horn)
4 Lateral ventricle
5 Caudate nucleus (head)
6 Thalamus (ventral lateral complex)
7 Globus pallidus
8 Choroid plexus
9 Anterior commissure
10 Thalamus (posterior lateral complex)
11 Internal capsule
12 Fornix (crus)
13 Putamen
14 Thalamus (pulvinar)
15 Posterior cerebral artery
16 Parahippocampal gyrus
17 Middle cerebral artery
18 Medial geniculate body

19 Orbital gyrus
20 Lingual gyrus
21 Sphenoidal bone (lesser wing)
22 Tentorium cerebelli
23 Optic nerve (II)
24 Hemisphere of cerebellum (anterior lobe)
25 Medial rectus muscle
26 Lateral geniculate body
27 Superior orbital fissure
28 Trochlear nerve (IV)
29 Oculomotor nerve (III)
30 Dentate nucleus
31 Middle cerebellar peduncle
32 Pons
33 Lateral ventricle (temporal horn)
34 Pontocerebellar cistern
35 Trigeminal nerve (V)
36 Internal carotid artery

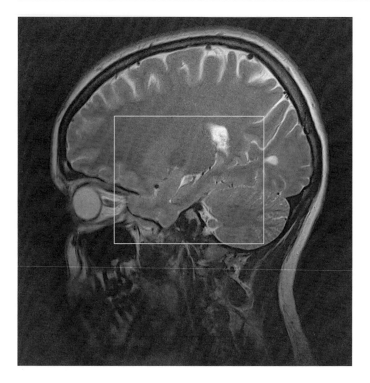

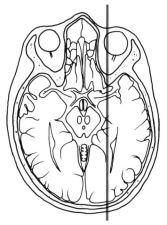

Frontal lobe
Temporal lobe
Parietal lobe
Occipital lobe
Cerebellum

1 Frontal bone and coronal suture
2 Parietal bone
3 Superior frontal gyrus
4 Postcentral gyrus
5 Caudate nucleus (body)
6 Precentral gyrus
7 Thalamus
8 Central sulcus

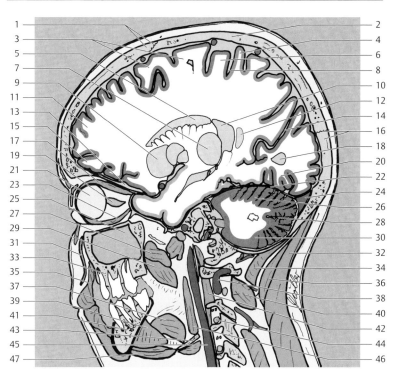

9 Basal nuclei
10 Lateral ventricle
11 Middle frontal gyrus
12 Corpus callosum
    (major forceps)
13 Roof of orbit
14 Parieto-occipital sulcus
15 Orbital gyrus
16 Occipital bone and lambdoid
    suture
17 Superior rectus muscle
18 Lateral ventricle (occipital
    horn)
19 Optic nerve (II)
20 Medial occipitotemporal gyrus
21 Eyeball
22 Tentorium cerebelli
23 Inferior rectus muscle
24 Transverse sinus
25 Maxillary sinus
26 Anterior lobe of cerebellum

27 Levator veli palatini muscle
28 Horizontal fissure
29 Medial pterygoid muscle
30 Posterior lobe of cerebellum
31 Levator labii superioris muscle
32 Splenius capitis muscle
33 Maxilla
34 Rectus capitis posterior major muscle
35 Orbicularis oris muscle
36 Semispinalis capitis muscle
37 Hypoglossus muscle
38 Vertebral artery
39 Mylohyoid muscle
40 Obliquus capitis inferior muscle
41 Mandible
42 Longus capitis muscle
43 Hyoid bone
44 Spinal nerve root C3
45 Internal carotid artery
46 Middle constrictor muscle of pharynx
47 Digastric muscle

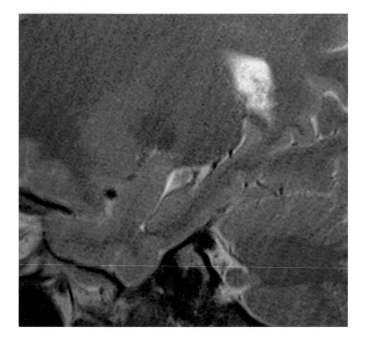

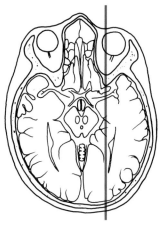

Frontal lobe
Temporal lobe
Parietal lobe
Occipital lobe
Cerebellum

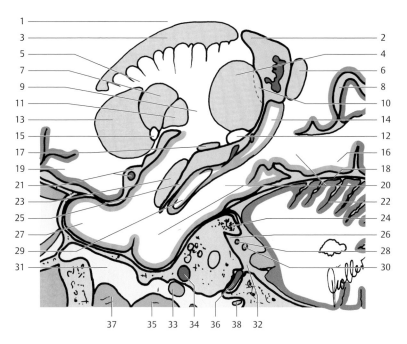

1 Corpus callosum (trunk)
2 Lateral ventricle (central part)
3 Caudate nucleus (body)
4 Thalamus (pulvinar)
5 Internal capsule (anterior limb)
6 Corpus callosum (major forceps)
7 Globus pallidus (lateral segment)
8 Parieto-occipital sulcus
9 Internal capsule (posterior limb)
10 Fornix (crus)
11 Globus pallidus (medial segment)
12 Lateral geniculate body
13 Putamen
14 Subiculum of hippocampus
15 Anterior commissure
16 Medial occipitotemporal gyrus
17 Optic tract
18 Tentorium cerebelli
19 Orbital gyrus
20 Parahippocampal gyrus

21 Middle cerebral artery in cistern of lateral cerebral fossa
22 Hemisphere of cerebellum (anterior lobe)
23 Amygdaloid nucleus
24 Petrous pyramid
25 Lateral ventricle (temporal horn)
26 Internal acoustic meatus
27 Temporal pole
28 Facial nerve (VII)
29 Dentate gyrus
30 Vestibulocochlear (acoustic) nerve (VIII)
31 Infratemporal fossa
32 Pontocerebellar cistern
33 Pharyngotympanic tube (auditory tube)
34 Internal carotid artery (petrous part)
35 Elevator muscle of the soft palate
36 Internal jugular vein in the jugular foramen
37 Medial pterygoid muscle
38 Hypoglossal nerve (XII) in hypoglossal canal

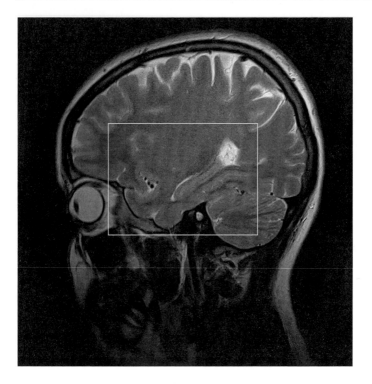

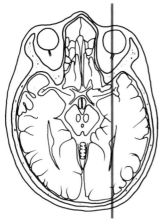

Frontal lobe
Temporal lobe
Parietal lobe
Occipital lobe
Cerebellum

1 Frontal bone and coronal suture
2 Parietal bone
3 Cerebral white matter (semioval
   center)
4 Precentral gyrus
5 Superior frontal gyrus
6 Postcentral gyrus
7 Basal ganglia

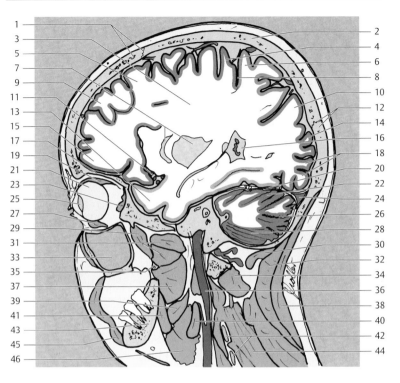

8 Central sulcus
9 Middle frontal gyrus
10 Precuneus
11 Insular arteries
12 Occipital bone and lambdoid suture
13 Temporal pole
14 Cuneus
15 Orbital gyrus
16 Lateral ventricle (occipital horn)
17 Roof of orbit
18 Occipital gyri
19 Superior rectus muscle
20 Tentorium cerebelli
21 Eyeball
22 Anterior lobe of cerebellum
23 Lateral rectus muscle
24 Transverse sinus
25 Lens
26 Horizontal fissure

27 Inferior rectus muscle
28 Posterior lobe of cerebellum
29 Temporal muscle
30 rectus capitis posterior major muscle
31 Lateral pterygoid muscle
32 Semispinalis capitis muscle
33 Maxillary sinus
34 Obliquus capitis inferior muscle
35 Pterygoid process, lateral plate
36 Internal carotid artery
37 Medial pterygoid muscle
38 Trapezius muscle
39 Styloglossus muscle
40 Digastric muscle
41 Mylohyoid muscle
42 Spinal nerve roots (cervical plexus)
43 Mandible
44 Levator scapulae muscle
45 Orbicularis oris muscle
46 Submandibular gland

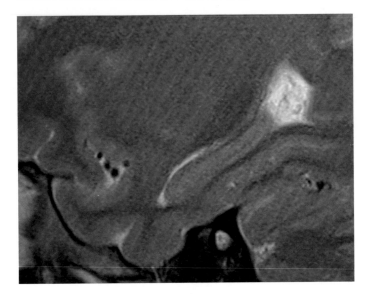

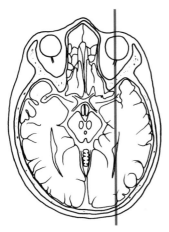

Frontal lobe
Temporal lobe
Parietal lobe
Occipital lobe
Cerebellum

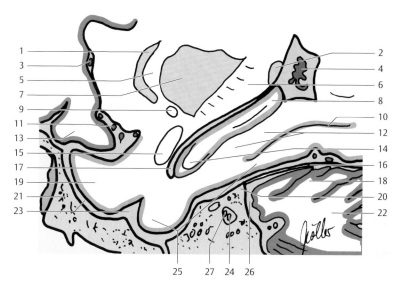

1 Claustrum
2 Caudate nucleus (tail)
3 Insular arteries
4 Lateral ventricle (central part) with choroid plexus
5 External capsule
6 Internal capsule
7 Putamen
8 Subiculum of hippocampus
9 Anterior commissure
10 Collateral sulcus
11 Middle cerebral artery
12 Parahippocampal gyrus
13 Orbital gyrus
14 Dentate gyrus
15 Amygdaloid nucleus
16 Tentorium cerebelli
17 Lateral ventricle (temporal horn)
18 Anterior lobe of cerebellum
19 Temporal lobe (temporal pole)
20 Petrous part of temporal bone (superior margin)
21 Sphenoidal bone (greater wing)
22 Cerebellum (cerebellar white matter)
23 Middle cranial fossa
24 Vestibulocochlear (acoustic) nerve (VIII) in Internal auditory meatus
25 Medial occipitotemporal gyrus
26 Pontocerebellar cistern
27 Facial nerve (VII) in Internal auditory meatus

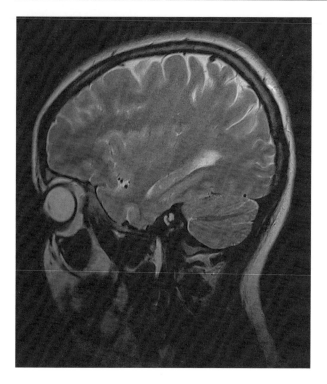

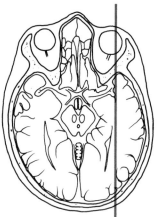

Frontal lobe
Temporal lobe
Parietal lobe
Occipital lobe
Cerebellum

1 Frontal bone and coronal suture
2 Parietal bone
3 Middle frontal gyrus
4 Precentral gyrus
5 Inferior frontal sulcus
6 Postcentral gyrus
7 Inferior frontal gyrus
8 Central sulcus
9 Insular gyri
10 Frontal operculum
11 Cistern of lateral cerebral fossa
     (insular cistern) and insular arteries

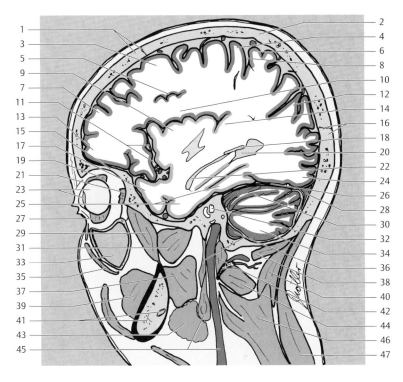

12 Precuneus
13 Orbital gyrus
14 Transverse temporal gyrus
15 Roof of orbit
16 Occipital bone and lambdoid
    suture
17 Temporal pole
18 Caudate nucleus (tail)
19 Levator palpebrae superioris
    muscle
20 Lateral ventricle
    (occipital horn)
21 Lateral rectus muscle
22 Lateral ventricle
    (temporal horn)
23 Eyeball and lens
24 Occipital gyri
25 Medial occipitotemporal gyrus
26 Tentorium cerebelli
27 Inferior oblique muscle
28 Transverse sinus
29 Temporal muscle

30 Anterior lobe of cerebellum
31 Lateral pterygoid muscle
32 Internal acoustic meatus
33 Maxillary sinus
34 Posterior lobe of cerebellum
35 Orbicularis oculi muscle
36 Sigmoid sinus and stylopharyngeus
    muscle
37 Medial pterygoid muscle
38 Rectus capitis posterior major muscle
39 Buccinator muscle
40 Semispinalis capitis muscle
41 Mandible and mandibular canal
    (inferior alveolar nerve)
42 Atlas (transverse process) and rectus
    capitis lateralis muscle
43 Submandibular gland
44 Obliquus capitis inferior muscle
45 Internal jugular vein and digastric
    muscle
46 Levator scapulae muscle
47 Splenius capitis muscle

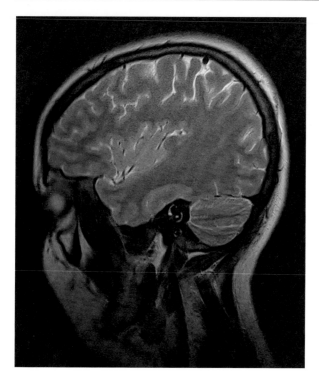

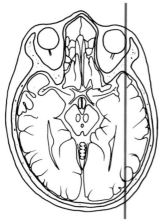

Frontal lobe
Temporal lobe
Parietal lobe
Occipital lobe
Cerebellum

1 Frontal bone and coronal
   suture
2 Parietal bone
3 Middle frontal gyrus
4 Precentral gyrus
5 Inferior frontal sulcus
6 Postcentral gyrus and
   postcentral sulcus
7 Insular gyri
8 Central sulcus

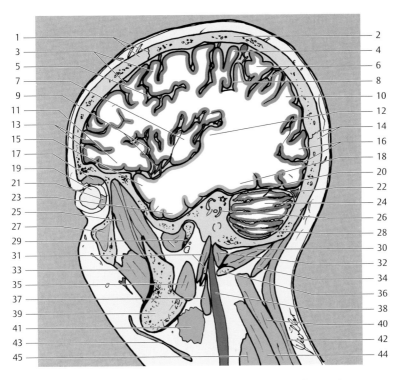

9   Cistern of lateral cerebral fossa
    (insular cistern) and insular
    arteries
10 Angular gyrus
11 Orbital gyrus
12 Transverse temporal gyrus
13 Inferior frontal gyrus
14 Occipital bone and lambdoid
    suture
15 Superior temporal gyrus
16 Occipital gyri
17 Lacrimal gland
18 Inferior temporal gyrus
19 Eyeball
20 Tentorium cerebelli
21 Lateral rectus muscle
22 Transverse sinus
23 Temporal pole and middle
    temporal gyrus
24 Anterior lobe of cerebellum
25 Temporal muscle

26 Posterior semicircular canal
27 Maxillary sinus
28 Posterior lobe of cerebellum
29 Lateral pterygoid muscle and head
    of mandible
30 Obliquus capitis superior muscle
31 Styloid muscle and styloid process
32 Rectus capitis lateralis muscle
33 Buccinator muscle
34 Semispinalis capitis muscle
35 Medial pterygoid muscle
36 Atlas, transverse process
37 Digastric muscle, posterior belly
38 Internal jugular vein
39 Mandible
40 Levator scapulae muscle
41 Submandibular gland
42 Splenius capitis muscle
43 Platysma
44 Splenius cervicis muscle
45 Scalenus posterior muscle

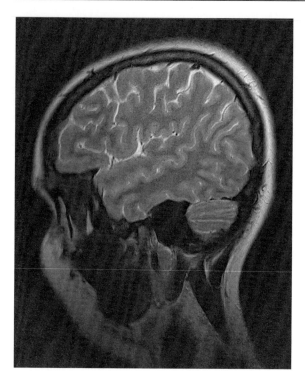

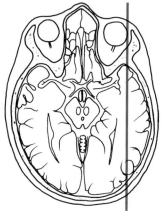

Frontal lobe
Temporal lobe
Parietal lobe
Cerebellum

1 Frontal bone and coronal suture
2 Parietal bone
3 Middle frontal gyrus
4 Precentral gyrus
5 Inferior frontal sulcus
6 Postcentral gyrus and
  postcentral sulcus

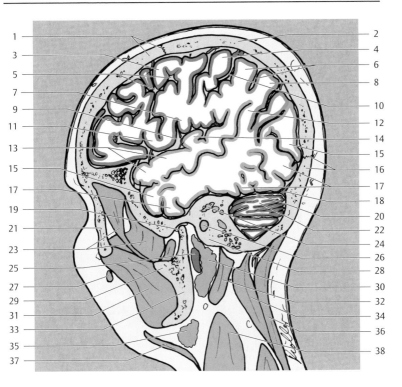

7 Inferior frontal gyrus, insular cortex
8 Supramarginal gyrus
9 Lateral sulcus
10 Central sulcus
11 Inferior frontal gyrus, opercular part
12 Angular gyrus
13 Superior temporal gyrus
14 Transverse temporal gyrus
15 Middle temporal gyrus
16 Occipital bone and lambdoid suture
17 Inferior temporal gyrus
18 Transverse sinus
19 Head of mandible
20 Tentorium cerebelli
21 Zygomatic bone
22 Posterior lobe of cerebellum
23 Temporal muscle
24 Mastoid antrum
25 Retromandibular vein
26 External acoustic meatus
27 Zygomatic muscle
28 Mastoid process
29 Coronoid process
30 Parotid gland
31 Masseter muscle
32 Digastric muscle, posterior belly
33 Mandible (ramus)
34 Semispinalis capitis muscle
35 Submandibular gland
36 Splenius capitis muscle
37 Platysma
38 Sternocleidomastoid muscle

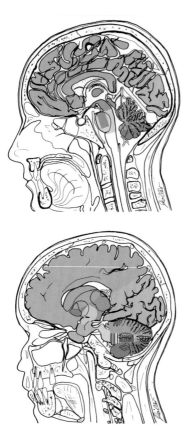
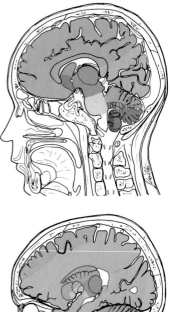
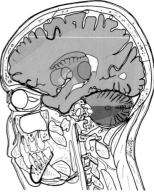

Anterior cerebral artery

Terminal branches

Central branches (striate arteries including distal medial striate artery)

Middle cerebral artery

Terminal branches

Central branches (striate branches)

Posterior cerebral artery

Terminal branches

Central branches (including the posterior communicating artery)

Basilar artery

Anteromedial and anterolateral paramedian branches

Circumferential arteries and lateral and dorsal paramedian branches

Superior cerebellar artery

Anterior superior cerebellar artery

Boundary region

Posterior inferior cerebellar artery

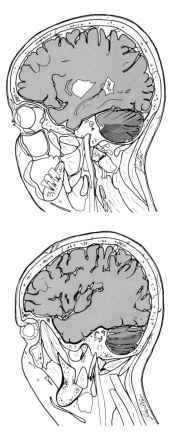
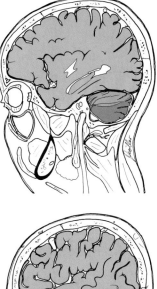
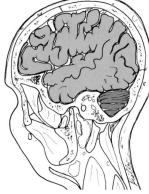

Middle cerebral artery
- Terminal branches
- Central branches (striate branches)

Posterior cerebral artery
- Terminal branches

- Anterior choroidal artery

- Superior cerebellar artery
- Anterior superior cerebellar artery
- Posterior inferior cerebellar artery

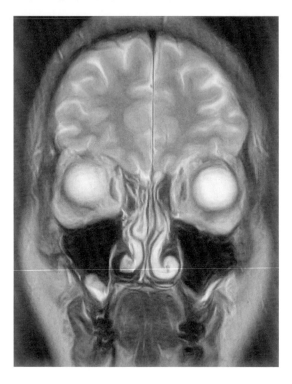

Frontal lobe

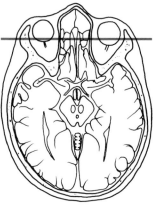

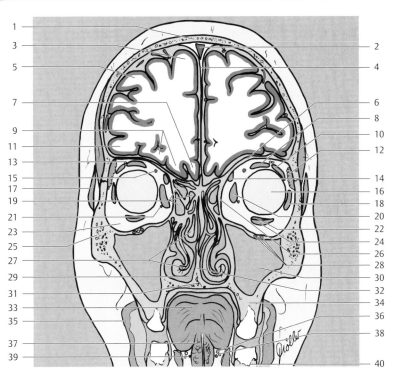

1 Frontal bone
2 Superior sagittal sinus
3 Superior frontal gyrus
4 Falx cerebri
5 Middle frontal gyrus
6 Roof of orbit
7 Straight gyrus
8 Levator palpebrae superioris
  muscle
9 Orbital gyri
10 Superior rectus muscle
11 Inferior frontal gyrus
12 Lacrimal gland
13 Supraorbital nerve
14 Superior oblique muscle
15 Superior ophthalmic vein
16 Eyeball
17 Orbicularis oculi muscle
18 Lateral rectus muscle
19 Ethmoidal cells
20 Medial rectus muscle

21 Ophthalmic artery
22 Inferior rectus muscle
23 Orbit (retrobulbar fat)
24 Inferior oblique muscle
25 Zygomatic bone
26 Orbital plate
27 Middle and inferior nasal conchas
28 Infraorbital artery, vein,
   and nerve
29 Nasal sinus
30 Maxillary sinus
31 Hard palate
32 Nasal septum
33 Tongue
34 Maxilla (alveolar process)
35 Depressor anguli oris muscle
36 Lingual nerve
37 Genioglossus muscle
38 Hypoglossal nerve (XII)
39 Submandibular duct
40 Body of mandible

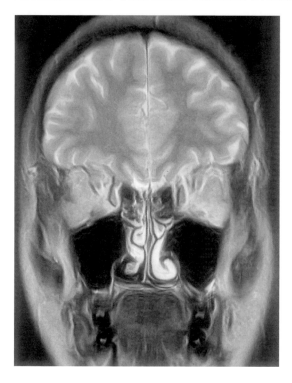

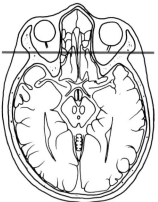

Frontal lobe

1 Frontal bone
2 Superior sagittal sinus
3 Superior frontal gyrus
4 Falx cerebri
5 Middle frontal gyrus
6 Longitudinal cerebral
7 Cingulate gyrus

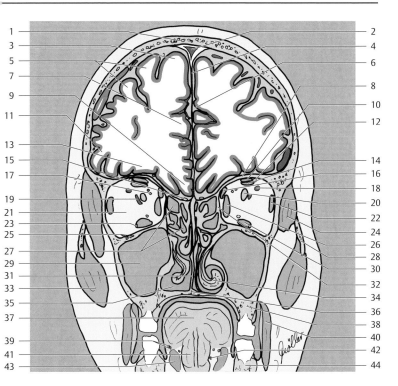

8 Roof of orbit
9 Straight gyrus
10 Levator palpebrae superioris muscle
11 Inferior frontal gyrus
12 Supraorbital nerve
13 Orbital gyri
14 Superior rectus muscle
15 Olfactory bulb
16 Superior oblique muscle
17 Nasociliary nerve
18 Superior ophthalmic vein
19 Ophthalmic artery
20 Optic nerve (II)
21 Orbit (retrobulbar fat)
22 Lateral rectus muscle
23 Oculomotor nerve (III), inferior part
24 Temporal muscle
25 Infraorbital nerve, artery, and vein

26 Medial rectus muscle
27 Ethmoidal cells
28 Zygomatic bone
29 Maxillary sinus
30 Inferior rectus muscle
31 Nasal septum
32 Orbital plate
33 Masseter muscle
34 Inferior nasal concha
35 Nasal cavity
36 Hard palate
37 Tongue
38 Maxilla (alveolar process)
39 Lingual nerve and hypoglossal nerve (XII)
40 Depressor anguli oris muscle
41 Genioglossus muscle
42 Submandibular duct
43 Submandibular gland
44 Body of mandible

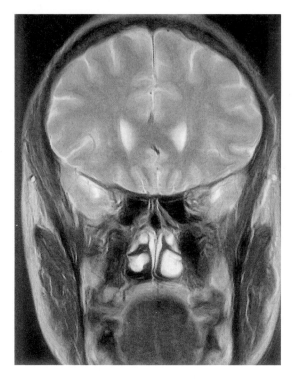

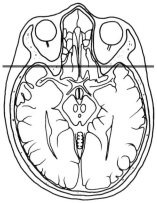

Frontal lobe
Temporal lobe

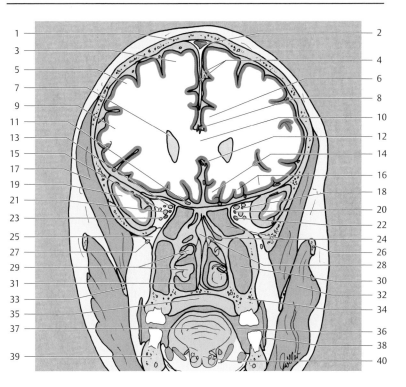

1 Frontal bone
2 Superior sagittal sinus
3 Superior frontal gyrus
4 Falx cerebri in interhemi-
   spheric fissure
5 Middle frontal gyrus
6 Cingulate gyrus
7 Lateral ventricle (frontal horn)
8 Pericallosal artery
9 Inferior frontal gyrus
10 Corpus callosum (genu)
11 Olfactory tract
12 Anterior cerebral artery
13 Optic nerve (II)
14 Straight gyrus
15 Oculomotor nerve (III)
16 Orbital gyri
17 Temporal muscle
18 Trochlear nerve (IV)
19 Temporal lobe (temporal pole)
20 Ophthalmic artery
21 Ophthalmic nerve (first division of
    trigeminal nerve)
22 Superior ophthalmic vein
23 Abducent nerve (VI)
24 Ethmoidal cells
25 Pterygopalatine fossa
26 Zygomatic arch
27 Maxillary nerve (second division of
    trigeminal nerve)
28 Nasal septum
29 Middle and inferior nasal conchas
30 Maxillary sinus
31 Nasal sinus
32 Masseter muscle
33 Ramus of mandible
34 Maxilla (alveolar process)
35 Soft palate
36 Oral cavity
37 Tongue
38 Buccinator muscle
39 Body of mandible
40 Genioglossus muscle

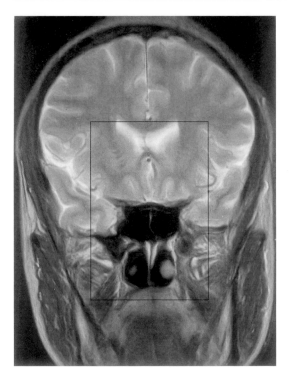

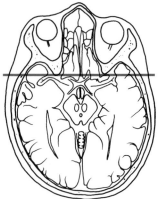

Frontal lobe

Temporal lobe

1 Frontal bone
2 Superior sagittal sinus
3 Superior frontal gyrus
4 Falx cerebri in Longitudinal cerebral
5 Middle frontal gyrus
6 Cingulate sulcus
7 Pericallosal artery

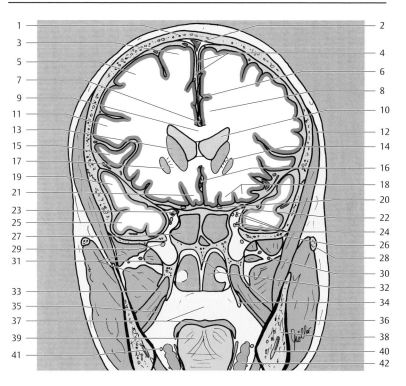

8 Cingulate gyrus
9 Corpus callosum (trunk)
10 Lateral ventricle (frontal horn)
11 Inferior frontal gyrus
12 Temporal muscle
13 Head of caudate nucleus
14 Internal capsule (anterior limb)
15 Frontal operculum
16 Anterior cerebral artery
17 Putamen
18 Orbital gyri
19 Superior temporal gyrus
20 Olfactory tract
21 Straight gyrus
22 Sphenoidal bone (lesser wing)
23 Optic nerve (II)
24 Trochlear (IV), oculomotor (III), ophthalmic (first division of trigeminal), and abducent (VI) nerves
25 Middle temporal gyrus

26 Temporal bone
27 Sphenoidal sinus
28 Zygomatic arch
29 Maxillary nerve in pterygopalatine fossa
30 Maxillary artery
31 Lateral pterygoid muscle in infra-temporal fossa
32 Nasal septum and sinus
33 Medial pterygoid muscle
34 Pterygoid process (medial and lateral plates)
35 Tensor veli palatini muscle
36 Masseter muscle
37 Soft palate and oral cavity
38 Ramus of mandible
39 Tongue
40 Inferior alveolar artery, vein, and nerve in mandibular canal
41 Lingual nerve
42 Submandibular gland

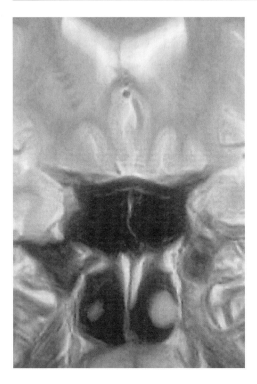

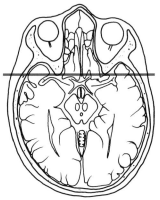

■ Frontal lobe
□ Temporal lobe

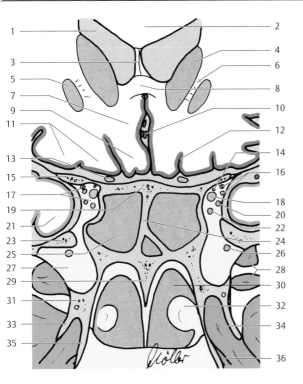

1 Lateral ventricle (frontal horn)
2 Corpus callosum (trunk)
3 Septum pellucidum
4 Head of caudate nucleus
5 Putamen
6 Internal capsule (anterior limb)
7 Subcallosal gyrus
8 Corpus callosum (genu)
9 Straight gyrus
10 Pericallosal artery
11 Orbital gyri
12 Olfactory sulcus
13 Olfactory tract
14 Oculomotor nerve (III, superior branch)
15 Anterior clinoid process (sphenoidal bone, lesser wing)
16 Ophthalmic nerve (frontal, lacrimal, and nasociliary nerves) = superior branch of trigeminal nerve (V)
17 Superior orbital fissure
18 Optic nerve (II)
19 Sphenoid plane
20 Abducent nerve (VI)
21 Temporal pole
22 Oculomotor nerve (III), inferior branch
23 Sphenoidal bone, lesser wing
24 Septum of sphenoidal sinus
25 Sphenoidal sinus
26 Maxillary nerve in pterygopalatine fossa
27 Pterygopalatine fossa
28 Lateral pterygoid muscle
29 Vomer
30 Nasal sinus
31 Pterygoid process (sphenoidal bone)
32 Middle nasal concha
33 Pterygoid process (lateral plate)
34 Medial pterygoid muscle
35 Pterygoid process (medial plate)
36 Tensor veli palatini muscle

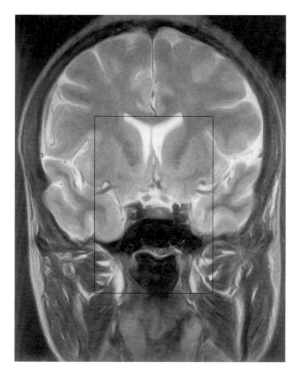

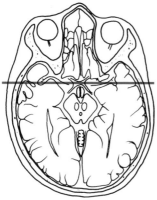

■ Frontal lobe
■ Temporal lobe

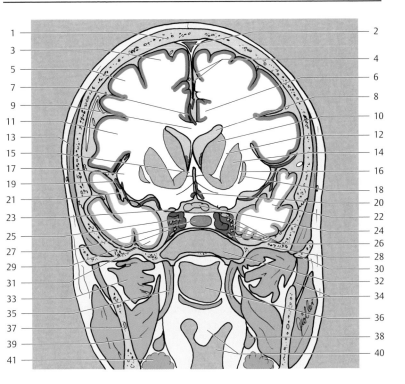

1 Frontal bone
2 Superior sagittal sinus
3 Superior frontal gyrus
4 Falx cerebri in
   Longitudinal cerebral
5 Middle frontal gyrus
6 Cingulate gyrus
7 Pericallosal artery
8 Lateral ventricle (frontal horn)
9 Corpus callosum (genu)
10 Head of caudate nucleus
11 Inferior frontal gyrus
12 Internal capsule (anterior limb)
13 Temporal muscle
14 Putamen
15 Subcallosal gyrus
16 External capsule
17 Insula
18 Claustrum
19 Insular arteries
20 Anterior cerebral artery
21 Lateral sulcus
22 Superior temporal gyrus
23 Olfactory tract
24 Optic chiasm
25 Internal carotid artery (syphon)
26 Trochlear (IV), oculomotor (III),
   ophthalmic, and abducent (V) nerves
27 Pituitary gland
28 Temporal bone
29 Cavernous sinus
30 Zygomatic bone
31 Middle temporal gyrus
32 Sphenoidal sinus
33 Lateral pterygoid muscle
34 Masseter muscle
35 Tensor veli palatini muscle
36 Nasopharynx
37 Ramus of mandible
38 Styloglossus muscle
39 Medial pterygoid muscle
40 Uvula and oropharynx
41 Submandibular gland

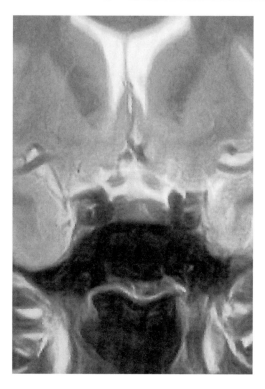

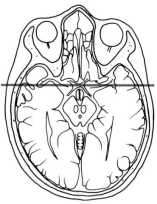

Temporal lobe

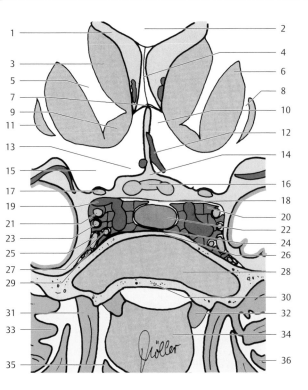

1 Lateral ventricle (frontal horn)
2 Corpus callosum (trunk)
3 Head of caudate nucleus
4 Septum pellucidum
5 Internal capsule (anterior limb)
6 Putamen
7 Corpus callosum (rostrum)
8 External capsule
9 Nucleus acumbens
10 Subcallosal gyrus
11 Claustrum
12 Anterior cerebral artery
13 Straight gyrus
14 Chiasmatic cistern
15 Orbital gyri
16 Optic chiasm
17 Olfactory tract
18 Sellar diaphragm
19 Internal carotid artery (syphon)
20 Cavernous sinus
21 Oculomotor nerve (III)
22 Pituitary gland
23 Trochlear nerve (IV)
24 Inferior intercavernous sinus
25 Ophthalmic nerve (V_1)
26 Floor of sella
27 Abducent nerve (VI)
28 Sphenoidal sinus
29 Maxillary nerve (V_2)
30 Sphenoidal bone (body)
31 Tensor veli palatini muscle
32 Pharyngotympanic tube
   (auditory tube)
33 Lateral pterygoid muscle
34 Nasopharynx
35 Levator veli palatini muscle
36 Medial pterygoid muscle

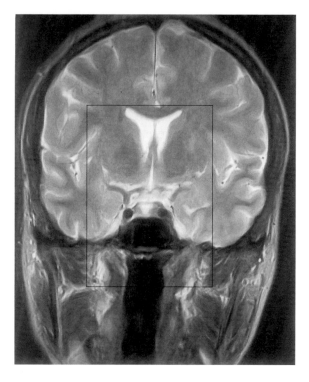

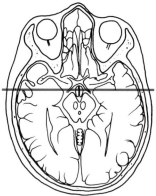

Frontal lobe
Temporal lobe

1 Frontal bone
2 Superior sagittal sinus
3 Falx cerebri in Longitudinal cerebral
4 Superior frontal gyrus
5 Pericallosal artery
6 Middle frontal gyrus
7 Corpus callosum (genu)

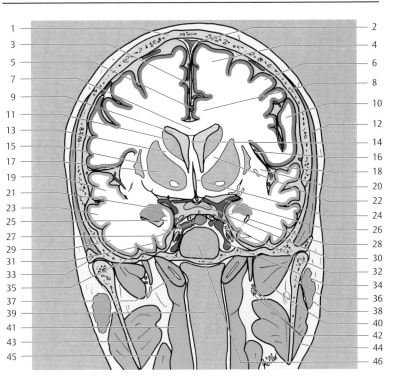

8 Cingulate gyrus
9 Lateral ventricle (frontal horn)
10 Inferior frontal gyrus
11 Head of caudate nucleus
12 Temporal muscle
13 External capsule
14 Septum pellucidum
15 Claustrum
16 Insular arteries
17 Putamen
18 Lateral sulcus
19 Superior temporal gyrus
20 Insula
21 Amygdaloid body
22 Internal capsule (anterior limb)
23 Middle temporal gyrus
24 Longitudinal cerebral
25 Hippocampus
26 Middle cerebral artery
27 Pituitary gland
28 Lateral ventricle (temporal horn)

29 Inferior temporal gyrus
30 Optic chiasm
31 Parahippocampal gyrus
32 Trochlear (IV), oculomotor (III) and abducent (VI) nerves, trigeminal ganglion
33 Temporal bone (zygomatic process)
34 Internal carotid artery (syphon)
35 Lateral occipitotemporal gyrus
36 Head of mandible
37 Pharyngotympanic tube (auditory tube)
38 Parotid gland
39 Pharynx
40 Lateral pterygoid muscle
41 Superior constrictor muscle of pharynx
42 Mandibular artery, vein, and nerve
43 Medial pterygoid muscle
44 Masseter muscle
45 Styloglossus muscle
46 Sphenoidal sinus

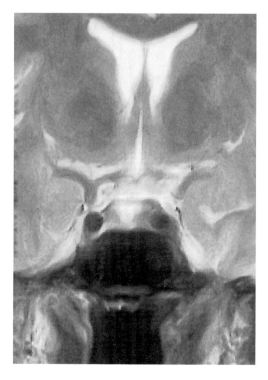

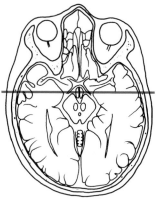

Temporal lobe

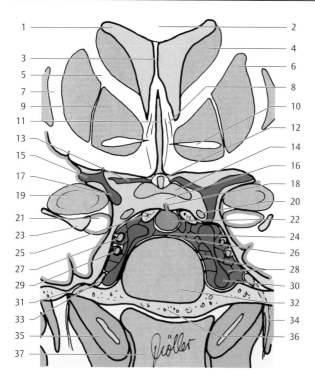

1 Lateral ventricle (frontal horn)
2 Corpus callosum (trunk)
3 Septum pellucidum
4 Head of caudate nucleus
5 Internal capsule (anterior limb)
6 Putamen
7 External capsule
8 Precommissural fornix
9 Globus pallidus
10 Anterior commissure
11 Longitudinal cerebral
12 Supraoptic recess
13 Anterior cerebral artery (A1 segment)
14 Optic chiasm
15 Middle cerebral artery
16 Suprasellar cistern
17 Internal carotid artery
18 Infundibulum
19 Amygdaloid body
20 Oculomotor nerve (III)
21 Hippocampus
22 Pituitary gland
23 Lateral ventricle (temporal horn)
24 Inferior intercavernous sinus
25 Posterior clinoid process
26 Floor of sella
27 Trochlear nerve (IV)
28 Cavernous sinus
29 Abducent nerve (VI), trigeminal ganglion
30 Internal carotid artery (syphon)
31 Foramen ovale
32 Sphenoidal sinus
33 Trigeminal (V) ganglion
34 Mandibular nerve (V_3)
35 Pharyngotympanic (auditory) tube
36 Sphenoidal bone (body)
37 Nasopharynx

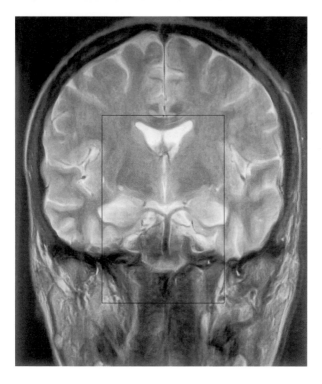

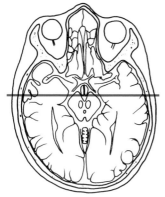

Frontal lobe
Temporal lobe
Parietal lobe

1 Frontal bone
2 Superior sagittal sinus
3 Falx cerebri in Longitudinal cerebral
4 Superior frontal gyrus
5 Cingulate gyrus
6 Middle frontal gyrus
7 Corpus callosum (trunk)
8 Cerebral white matter (semioval center)

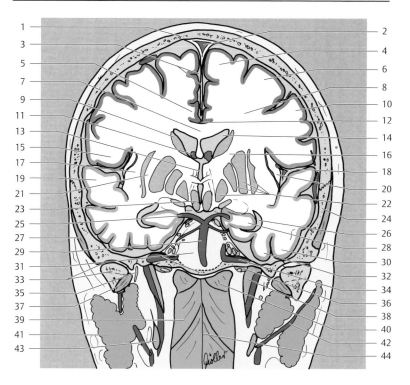

9 Caudate nucleus (body)
10 Inferior frontal gyrus
11 Interventricular foramen
12 Pericallosal artery
13 Third ventricle
14 Lateral ventricle (frontal horn)
15 Frontal operculum
16 Internal capsule (genu)
17 Extreme capsule
18 Lateral sulcus
19 Superior temporal gyrus
20 Insula
21 External capsule
22 Basal nuclei
   (lentiform nucleus)
23 Mammillary body and
   hypothalamus
24 Temporal bone
25 Posterior cerebral artery
26 Lateral ventricle (temporal
   horn)

27 Temporal muscle
28 Hippocampus
29 Basilar artery
30 Middle temporal gyrus
31 Occipital bone (clivus)
32 Lateral occipitotemporal gyrus
33 Head of mandible and
   temporomandibular joint
34 Internal carotid artery (syphon)
35 Mandibular nerve
36 Pharyngotympanic (auditory) tube
37 Lateral pterygoid muscle
38 Levator veli palatini muscle
39 Constrictor muscle of pharynx
   (superior, middle, and inferior)
40 Pharyngobasilar fascia
41 Parotid gland
42 External carotid artery
43 Stylopharyngeus muscle
44 Pharyngeal raphe

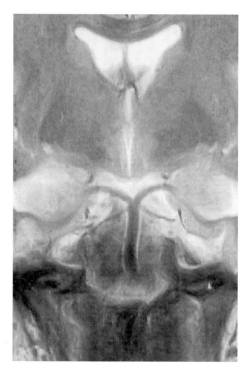

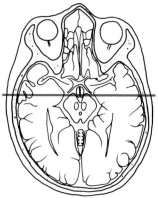

Temporal lobe

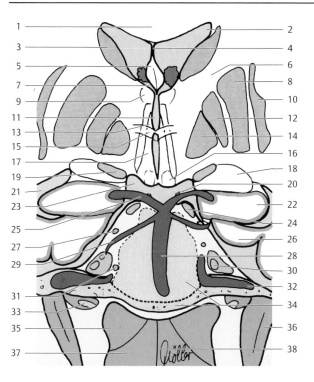

1 Corpus callosum (trunk)
2 Lateral ventricle (frontal horn)
3 Body of caudate nucleus
4 Septum pellucidum
5 Fornix (body)
6 Internal capsule (genu)
7 Interventricular foramen
8 Putamen
9 Thalamus (anterior ventral nucleus)
10 Claustrum
11 Third ventricle
12 Globus pallidus lateral segment
13 Fornix (column)
14 Globus pallidus medial segment
15 Anterior commissure
16 Mammillary body
17 Hypothalamus
18 Amygdaloid body
19 Optic tract
20 Posterior communicating artery
21 Lateral ventricle (temporal horn)
22 Hippocampus
23 Ambient cistern
24 Oculomotor nerve (III)
25 Posterior cerebral artery
26 Parahippocampal gyrus
27 Trochlear nerve (IV)
28 Basilar artery
29 Superior cerebellar artery
30 Trigeminal nerve (ganglion, V)
31 Abducent nerve (VI)
32 Internal carotid artery (syphon)
33 Pharyngotympanic (auditory) tube
34 Occipital bone (basilar part), clivus
35 Pharyngobasilar fascia
36 Levator veli palatini muscle
37 Superior constrictor muscle of pharynx
38 Pharyngeal raphe

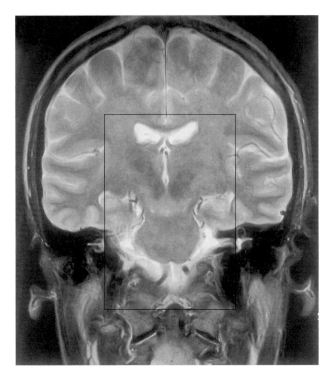

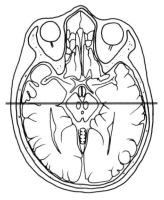

	Frontal lobe
	Temporal lobe
	Parietal lobe
	Mesencephalon
	Pons

1 Parietal bone
2 Superior sagittal sinus
3 Superior frontal gyrus
4 Falx cerebri
5 Central white matter (semioval center)
6 Cingulate gyrus
7 Precentral gyrus
8 Pericallosal artery
9 Central sulcus

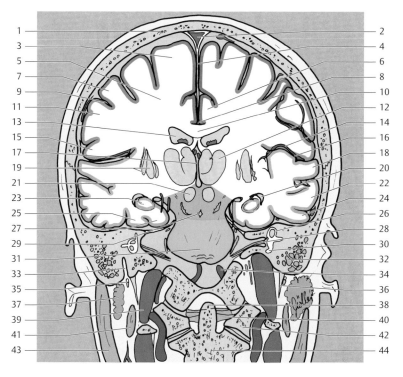

10 Corpus callosum (trunk)
11 Postcentral gyrus
12 Thalamus
13 Lateral ventricle
14 Insular arteries
15 Parietal operculum
16 Lateral sulcus
17 Third ventricle
18 Superior temporal gyrus
19 Basal nuclei (lentiform nucleus)
20 Lateral ventricle (temporal horn)
21 Red nucleus
22 Middle temporal gyrus
23 Hippocampus
24 Inferior temporal gyrus
25 Lateral occipitotemporal gyrus
26 Membranous semicircular canal (superior part)
27 Parahippocampal gyrus

28 Vestibulocochlear (VIII) and facial (VII) nerves in internal acoustic meatus
29 Interpeduncular cistern
30 Cochlea
31 Pons
32 Mastoid process with mastoid cells
33 Stylomastoid foramen
34 Vertebral artery
35 Facial nerve (VII)
36 Styloid process
37 Parotid gland
38 Dens
39 Internal jugular vein
40 Transverse ligament of atlas
41 Digastric muscle (posterior belly)
42 Atlas (lateral mass)
43 Sternocleidomastoid muscle
44 Axis

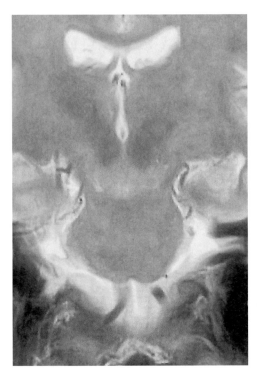

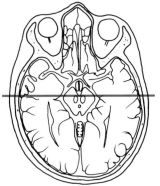

	Frontal lobe
	Temporal lobe
	Parietal lobe
	Mesencaphalon
	Pons
	Medulla oblongata

1 Corpus callosum (trunk)
2 Pericallosal artery
3 Caudate nucleus (body)
4 Lateral ventricle
5 Fornix (crus)
6 Internal cerebral vein
7 Thalamus (lateral dorsal nucleus)
8 Internal capsule (posterior limb)

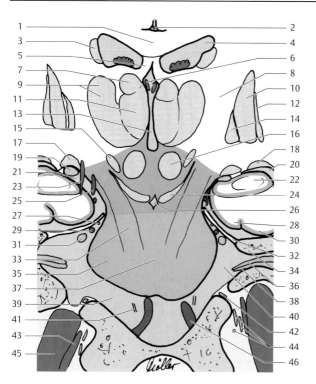

 9 Thalamus (ventral lateral complex)
10 Putamen
11 Thalamus (medial nuclei)
12 Claustrum
13 Third ventricle
14 Globus pallidus
15 Subthalamic nucleus
16 Red nucleus
17 Lateral geniculate body
18 Caudate nucleus (tail)
19 Optic tract
20 Lateral ventricle (temporal horn)
21 Ambient cistern
22 Hippocampus
23 Basal vein
24 Substantia nigra
25 Posterior cerebral artery
26 Interpeduncular cistern
27 Trochlear nerve (IV)
28 Parahippocampal gyrus

29 Superior cerebellar artery
30 Lateral occipitotemporal gyrus
31 Trigeminal nerve (V)
32 Tentorium cerebelli
33 Corticospinal tract
34 Petrous part of temporal bone
35 Middle cerebellar peduncle
36 Facial nerve (VII) in internal acoustic meatus
37 Pons
38 Vestibulocochlear nerve (VIII) in internal acoustic meatus
39 Prepontine cistern
40 Pontocerebellar cistern
41 Abducent nerve (VI)
42 Glossopharyngeal nerve (IX)
43 Vertebral vein
44 Vagus nerve (X), accessory nerve (XI), hypoglossal nerve (XII)
45 Internal jugular vein
46 Vertebral artery

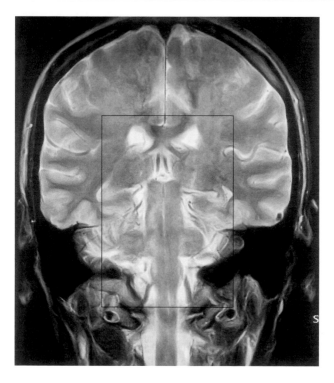

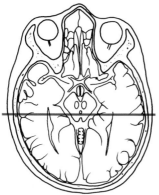

Frontal lobe
Temporal lobe
Parietal lobe
Cerebellum
Mesencephalon
Pons
Medulla oblongata

1 Parietal bone
2 Superior sagittal sinus
3 Superior frontal gyrus
4 Precentral gyrus
5 Paracentral lobe
6 Central sulcus
7 Falx cerebri
8 Postcentral gyrus
9 Cingulate gyrus

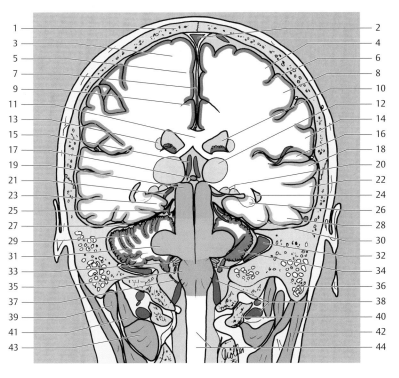

10 Lateral ventricle
11 Corpus callosum
12 Thalamus
13 Caudate nucleus
14 Supramarginal gyrus
15 Internal cerebral vein
16 Transverse temporal gyrus
17 Pineal body
18 Superior temporal gyrus
19 Cranial colliculus
20 Medial geniculate body and lateral geniculate body
21 Occipital artery
22 Middle temporal gyrus
23 Parahippocampal gyrus
24 Lateral ventricle (temporal horn)
25 Superior cerebellar artery
26 Hippocampus
27 Tentorium cerebelli
28 Inferior temporal gyrus
29 Anterior lobe of cerebellum
30 Lateral occipitotemporal gyrus
31 Middle cerebellar peduncle
32 Sigmoid sinus
33 Facial nerve (VII), vestibulocochlear nerve (VIII), glossopharyngeal nerve (IX)
34 Flocculus
35 Inferior olivary complex
36 Mastoid process with mastoid cells
37 Posterior inferior cerebellar artery
38 Vertebral artery and vein
39 Digastric muscle (posterior belly)
40 Atlas (lateral mass)
41 Obliquus capitis superior muscle
42 Sternocleidomastoid muscle
43 Obliquus capitis inferior muscle
44 Spinal cord with median fissure

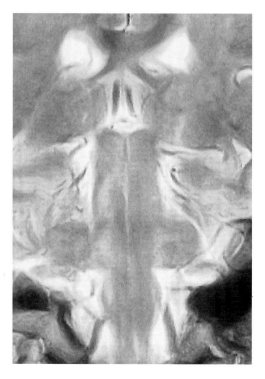

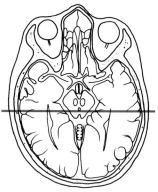

Temporal lobe
Cerebellum
Mesencephalon
Pons
Medulla oblongata

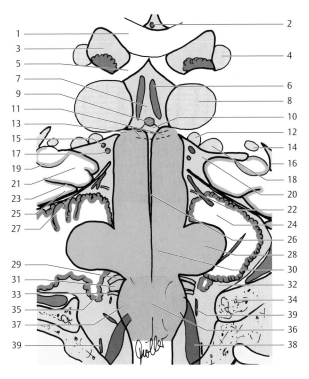

1 Corpus callosum (trunk)
2 Pericallosal artery
3 Lateral ventricle
4 Body of caudate nucleus
5 Fornix (crus)
6 Internal cerebral vein
7 Suprapineal recess
8 Thalamus (pulvinar)
9 Pineal body
10 Aqueduct of midbrain
11 Posterior commissure
12 Medial geniculate body
13 Cranial colliculus
14 Lateral geniculate body
15 Posterior cerebral artery
16 Caudate nucleus (tail)
17 Basal vein
18 Lateral ventricle (temporal horn)
19 Hippocampus
20 Ambient cistern
21 Parahippocampal gyrus
22 Trochlear nerve (IV)
23 Collateral sulcus
24 Anterior lobe of cerebellum
25 Lateral occipitotemporal gyrus
26 Aqueduct
27 Tentorium cerebelli
28 Middle cerebellar peduncle
29 Glossopharyngeal nerve (XI)
30 Pons
31 Vagus nerve (X)
32 Pontocerebellar cistern
33 Accessory nerve (XI)
34 Occipital bone
35 Flocculus
36 Medulla oblongata
37 Inferior olivary complex
38 Vertebral artery
39 Posterior inferior cerebellar artery

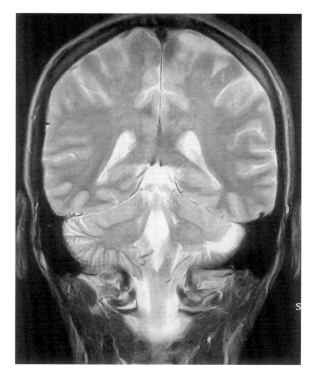

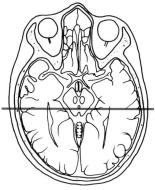

Frontal lobe
Temporal lobe
Parietal lobe
Cerebellum

1 Parietal bone
2 Superior sagittal sinus
3 Superior frontal gyrus
4 Falx cerebri
5 Precentral gyrus
6 Paracentral lobule
7 Central sulcus

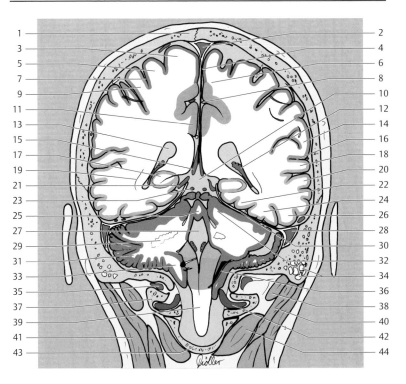

8 Precuneal artery
9 Postcentral gyrus
10 Quadrigeminal cistern
11 Precuneus
12 Choroid plexus
13 Lateral ventricle (collateral trigone)
14 Supramarginal gyrus
15 Internal cerebral vein
16 Lateral sulcus
17 Hippocampus
18 Superior temporal gyrus
19 Optic radiation
20 Middle temporal gyrus
21 Basal vein
22 Medial occipitotemporal gyrus
23 Superior cerebellar artery
24 Lateral occipitotemporal gyrus
25 Vermis of cerebellum

26 Inferior temporal gyrus
27 Fourth ventricle
28 Transverse sinus
29 Dentate nucleus
30 Tentorium cerebelli
31 Posterior lobe of cerebellum
32 Anterior lobe of cerebellum
33 Tonsil of cerebellum
34 Mastoid cells in mastoid process
35 Vertebral vein
36 Posterior inferior cerebellar artery
37 Atlas (lateral mass)
38 Obliquus capitis superior muscle
39 Spinal cord
40 Longus capitis muscle
41 Sternocleidomastoid muscle
42 Vertebral artery
43 Third cervical vertebra (arch)
44 Obliquus capitis inferior muscle

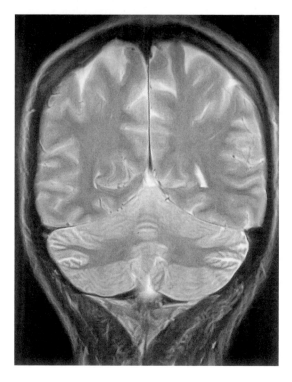

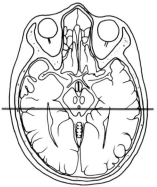

Frontal lobe
Temporal lobe
Parietal lobe
Cerebellum

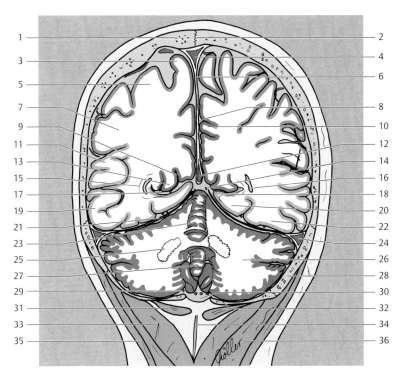

1 Parietal bone
2 Sagittal suture
3 Precentral gyrus
4 Superior sagittal sinus
5 Postcentral gyrus
6 Falx cerebri
7 Supramarginal gyrus
8 Longitudinal cerebral
9 Parieto-occipital sulcus
10 Precuneus
11 Middle temporal gyrus
12 Straight sinus
13 Cuneus
14 Superior cerebellar artery
15 Optic radiation
16 Lateral ventricle (occipital horn)
17 Calcarine sulcus
18 Striate cortex
19 Inferior temporal gyrus
20 Medial occipitotemporal gyrus
21 Tentorium cerebelli
22 Lateral occipitotemporal gyrus
23 Vermis of cerebellum
24 Transverse sinus
25 Dentate nucleus
26 Posterior lobe of cerebellum
27 Uvula of vermis
28 Temporal bone
29 Posterior inferior cerebellar artery
30 Cisterna magna
31 Rectus capitis posterior minor muscle
32 Occipital bone
33 Rectus capitis posterior major muscle
34 Nuchal ligament
35 Splenius capitis muscle
36 Semispinalis capitis muscle

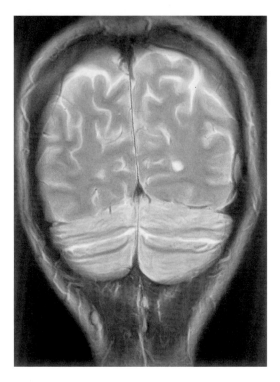

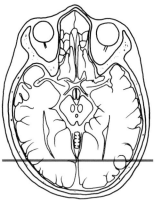

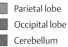

Parietal lobe

Occipital lobe

Cerebellum

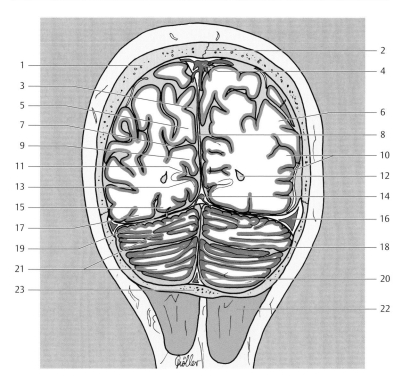

1 Parietal bone
2 Sagittal suture
3 Longitudinal cerebral
4 Superior sagittal sinus
5 Precuneus
6 Angular gyrus
7 Parieto-occipital sulcus
8 Falx cerebri
9 Cuneus
10 Occipital gyri
11 Calcarine sulcus
12 Lateral ventricle (occipital horn)
13 Striate cortex
14 Straight sinus
15 Medial occipitotemporal gyrus
16 Transverse sinus
17 Lateral occipitotemporal gyrus
18 Horizontal fissure
19 Tentorium cerebelli
20 Occipital sinus
21 Posterior lobe of cerebellum
22 Semispinalis capitis muscle
23 Occipital bone

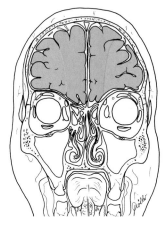

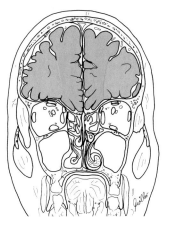

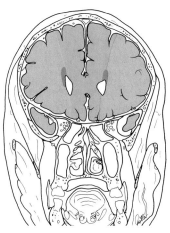

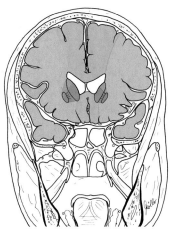

Anterior cerebral artery
Terminal branches
Central branches

Middle cerebral artery
Terminal branches
Central branches

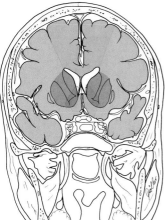
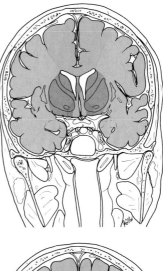
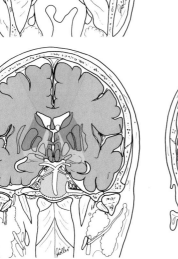
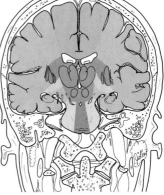

Anterior cerebral artery

 Terminal branches

Central branches (striate arteries including distal medial striate artery)

Middle cerebral artery

Terminal branches

Central branches (striate branches)

Posterior cerebral artery

 Terminal branches

Central branches (including posterior communicating artery)

 Anterior choroidal artery

Basilar artery

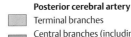 Anteromedial and anterolateral paramedian branches

Circumferential arteries and lateral and dorsal paramedian branches

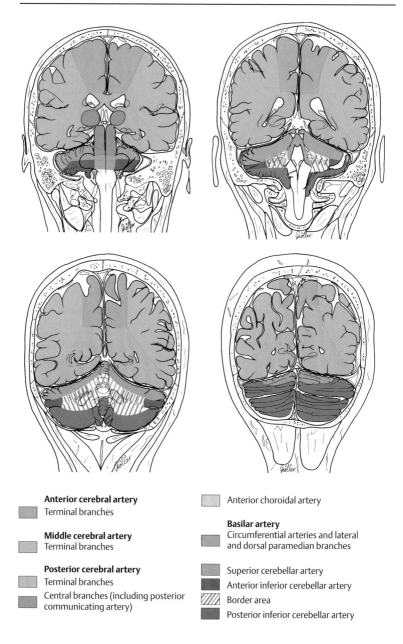

Anterior cerebral artery
Terminal branches

Middle cerebral artery
Terminal branches

Posterior cerebral artery
Terminal branches
Central branches (including posterior communicating artery)

Anterior choroidal artery

Basilar artery
Circumferential arteries and lateral and dorsal paramedian branches

Superior cerebellar artery
Anterior inferior cerebellar artery
Border area
Posterior inferior cerebellar artery

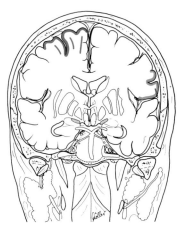
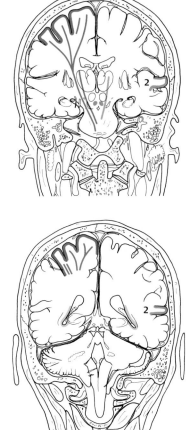
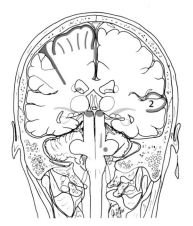

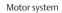 Motor system

Sensory system

Medial lemniscus

Spinothalamic tract

Mesencephalic nucleus of
trigeminal nerve

Oculomotor nucleus and
pathways

Optic tract

Speech center
(1 = motor, 2 = sensory)

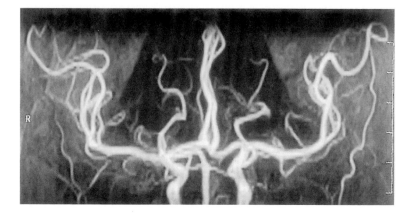

Frontal view

Anterior cerebral artery

Middle cerebral artery

Posterior cerebral artery

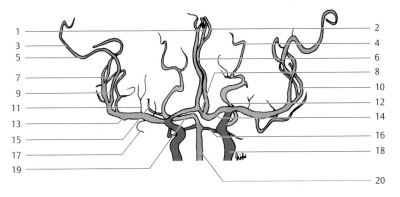

1 Callosomarginal artery
2 Pericallosal artery
3 Superior parietal artery
4 Posterior cerebral artery
   (parieto-occipital ramus)
5 Middle cerebral artery
   (opercular part, M3 segment)
6 Anterior cerebral artery
   (postcommunicating part)
7 Insular arteries
8 Anterior communicating
   artery
9 Middle cerebral artery
   (insular part, M2 segment)
10 Anterior temporal artery and
   middle temporal artery

11 Striate artery
12 Left posterior cerebral artery (from
   internal carotid artery, variant)
13 Middle cerebral artery (sphenoid
   part, M1 segment)
14 Anterior cerebral artery
   (precommunicating part)
15 Posterior cerebral artery (temporal
   and occipitotemporal branches)
16 Superior cerebellar artery
17 Polar temporal artery
18 Internal carotid artery
19 Right posterior cerebral artery
20 Basilar artery

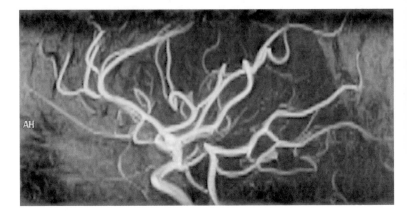

Lateral view

- [ ] Anterior cerebral artery
- [ ] Middle cerebral artery
- [ ] Posterior cerebral artery

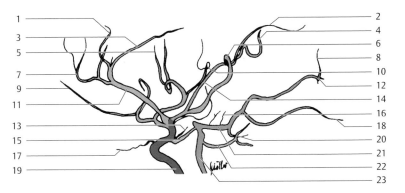

1 Callosomarginal artery
2 Parietal artery
3 Pericallosal artery
4 Artery of angular gyrus
5 Artery of precentral sulcus
6 Middle cerebral artery
(opercular part)
7 Polar frontal artery
8 Parieto-occipital artery
9 Medial frontobasal artery
10 Artery of central sulcus
11 Anterior cerebral artery
(postcommunicating segment,
A2 segment)

12 Medial occipital artery
13 Anterior choroidal artery
14 Middle cerebral artery (M2 segment)
15 Posterior communicating artery
16 Posteromedial central arteries
17 Ophthalmic artery
18 Occipitotemporal branch
19 Internal carotid artery
20 Posterior temporal artery
21 Posterior cerebral artery
22 Superior cerebellar artery
23 Basilar artery

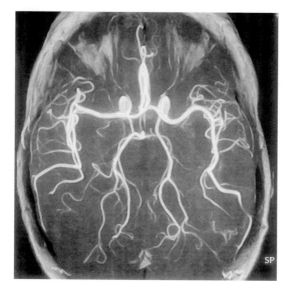

Cranial view

 Anterior cerebral artery

Middle cerebral artery

Posterior cerebral artery

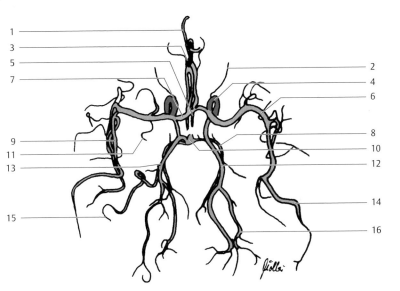

1 Anteromedial frontal branch of anterior cerebral artery
2 Ophthalmic artery
3 Anterior cerebral artery (postcommunicating part)
4 Internal carotid artery
5 Anterior communicating artery
6 Middle cerebral artery (sphenoid part)
7 Anterior cerebral artery (precommunicating part)
8 Superior cerebellar artery
9 Middle cerebral artery (insular part)
10 Basilar artery
11 Anterior choroidal artery
12 Left posterior cerebral artery (from internal carotid artery, variant)
13 Right posterior cerebral artery
14 Middle cerebral artery (opercular part)
15 Temporal artery
16 Parieto-occipital artery

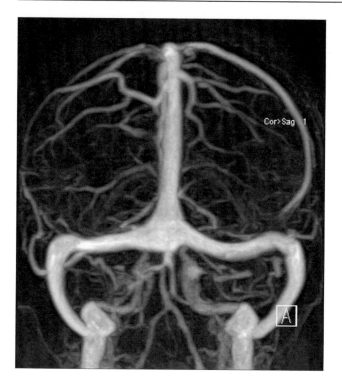

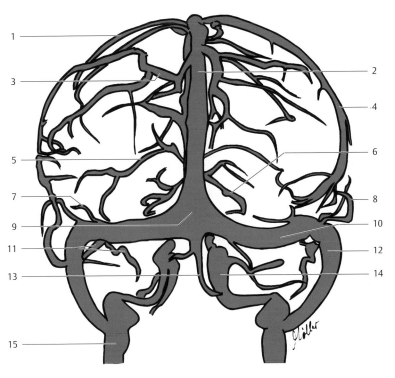

1 Superior cerebral veins
2 Superior sagittal sinus
3 Parietal veins
4 Superior anastomotic vein
  (Trolard)
5 Frontal veins
6 Basal vein
7 Middle cerebral veins (deep
  and superficial)

8 Sphenoparietal sinus
9 Confluence of sinuses
10 Transverse sinus
11 Superior veins of cerebellar
  hemisphere
12 Sigmoid sinus
13 Inferior of cerebellar hemisphere
14 Cavernous sinus
15 Internal jugular vein

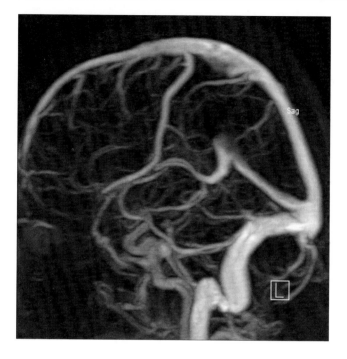

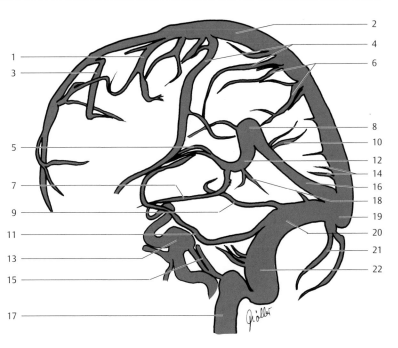

1   Precentral cerebellar veins
2   Superior sagittal sinus
3   Frontal veins
4   Superior cerebral veins
5   Internal cerebral veins
6   Parietal veins
7   Basal vein
8   Falcotentorial confluence
    of sinuses
9   Inferior anastomotic vein
    (Labbé)
10 Internal occipital vein
11 Superior petrosal sinus
12 Great cerebral vein
13 Cavernous sinus
14 Posterior cerebral veins
15 Inferior petrosal sinus
16 Straight sinus
17 Internal jugular vein
18 Superior veins of cerebellar
    hemisphere
19 Confluence of sinuses
20 Transverse sinus
21 Inferior veins of cerebellar
    hemisphere
22 Sigmoid sinus

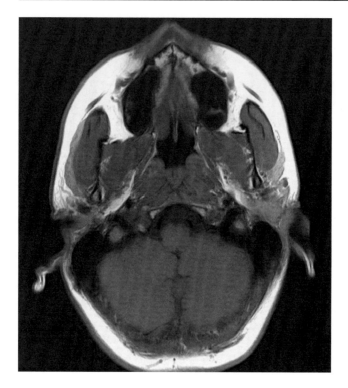

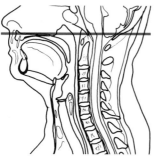

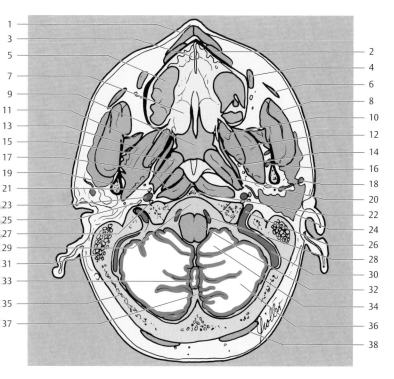

1 Orbicularis oris muscle
2 Levator labii superioris muscle
3 Maxilla (palatine process) and incisive canal
4 Levator anguli oris muscle
5 Maxillary sinus
6 Major zygomaticus muscle
7 Soft palate
8 Masseter muscle
9 Nasopharynx
10 Medial pterygoid muscle
11 Temporal muscle
12 Tensor veli palatini muscle
13 Lateral pterygoid muscle
14 Mandibular nerve (V₃)
15 Pharyngotympanic tube (auditory tube) (torus levatorius)
16 Maxillary artery
17 Longus capitis muscle
18 Retromandibular vein
19 Ramus of mandible
20 Levator veli palatini muscle
21 Glossopharyngeal nerve (IX)
22 Occipital bone, basilar part (basion)
23 Internal carotid artery
24 Parotid gland
25 Vagus nerve (X)
26 Internal jugular vein (superior bulb)
27 Hypoglossal nerve (XII)
28 Vertebral artery
29 Interpeduncular cistern
30 Sigmoid sinus
31 Mastoid cells
32 Medulla oblongata
33 Vermis
34 Tonsil of cerebellum
35 Occipital bone
36 Cerebellar hemisphere (posterior lobe)
37 Cisterna magna (posterior cerebellomedullary cistern)
38 Semispinalis capitis muscle

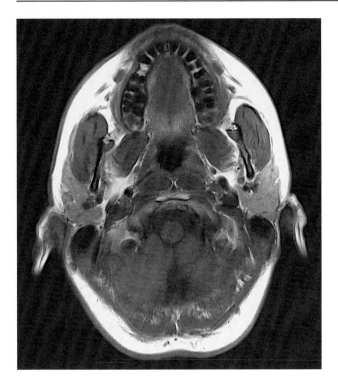

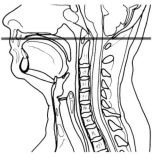

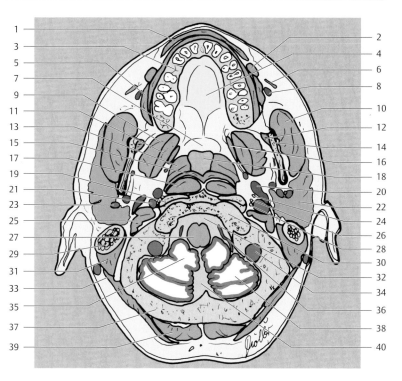

1 Orbicularis oris muscle
2 Levator anguli oris muscle
3 Maxilla (alveolar process)
4 Hard palate
5 Buccinator muscle
6 Zygomaticus muscle
7 Soft palate
8 Facial artery
9 Lateral pterygoid muscle
10 Masseter muscle
11 Medial pterygoid muscle
12 Temporal muscle
13 Levator veli palatini muscle
14 Ramus of mandible
15 Splenius capitis muscle
16 Tensor veli palatini muscle
17 Longus capitis muscle
18 Nasopharynx
19 Anterior arch of atlas
20 Internal carotid artery
21 Internal jugular vein
22 Parotid gland

23 Retromandibular vein
24 Vagus nerve (X)
25 Rectus capitis lateralis muscle
26 Hypoglossal nerve (XII)
27 Medulla oblongata
28 Accessory nerve (XI)
29 Mastoid cells (mastoid process)
30 Occipital bone, basilar part
  (basion)
31 Digastric muscle (posterior belly)
32 Interpeduncular cistern
33 Splenius capitis muscle
34 Condylar canal with emissary veins
35 Tonsil of cerebellum
36 Vertebral artery
37 Occipital bone
38 Cerebellar hemisphere
  (posterior lobe)
39 Semispinalis capitis muscle
40 Cisterna magna (posterior
  cerebellomedullary cistern)

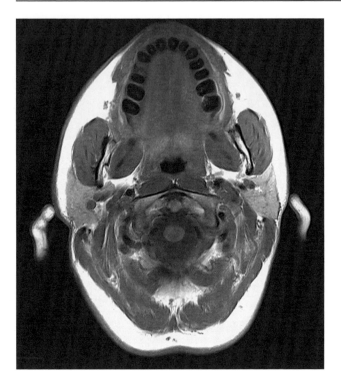

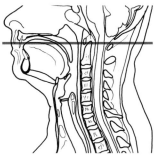

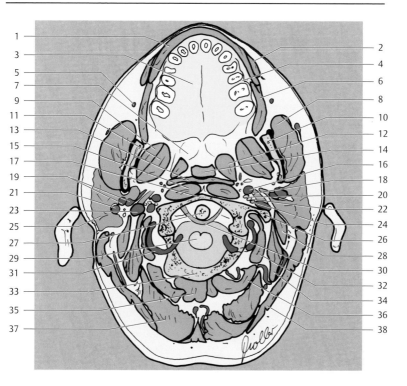

1 Orbicularis oris muscle
2 Levator anguli oris muscle
3 Hard palate
4 Maxilla (alveolar process)
5 Facial artery
6 Buccinator muscle
7 Soft palate
8 Masseter muscle
9 Lateral pterygoid muscle
10 Ramus of mandible
11 Medial pterygoid muscle
12 Tensor veli palatini muscle
13 Superior constrictor muscle of pharynx
14 Pharynx
15 Longus capitis muscle
16 Internal carotid artery
17 Atlas (anterior arch)
18 Glossopharyngeal nerve (IX)
19 Maxillary artery and vein
20 Vagus nerve (X)
21 Retromandibular vein
22 Hypoglossal nerve (XII)
23 Stylopharyngeus muscle
24 Accessory nerve (XI)
25 Parotid gland
26 Atlas, transverse process
27 Dens of axis
28 Digastric muscle (posterior belly)
29 Medulla oblongata
30 Transverse ligament of atlas
31 Vertebral artery
32 Rectus capitis lateralis muscle
33 Atlas, posterior arch
34 Obliquus capitis superior muscle
35 Rectus capitis posterior minor muscle
36 Obliquus capitis inferior muscle
37 Semispinalis capitis muscle
38 Splenius capitis muscle

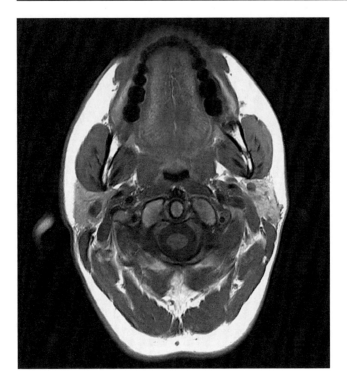

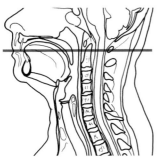

1 Upper lip
2 Incisors (1 and 2 left)
3 Orbicularis oris muscle
4 Canine tooth (3 left)
5 Levator anguli oris muscle
6 Premolar teeth (4 and 5 left)

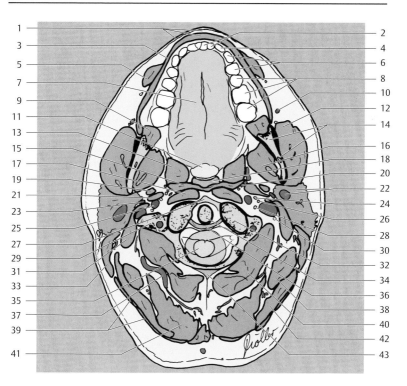

7 Tongue
8 Molar teeth (6,7 and 8)
9 Buccinator muscle
10 Facial artery
11 Uvula
12 Masseter muscle
13 Tensor veli palatini muscle
14 Ramus of mandible with alveolar canal
15 Superior constrictor muscle of pharynx
16 Medial pterygoid muscle
17 Longus capitis muscle
18 Oropharynx
19 Styloglossus muscle
20 Pharyngeal venous plexus
21 Stylopharyngeus muscle
22 Parotid gland and retromandibular vein
23 Maxillary artery
24 Glossopharyngeal nerve (IX)

25 Internal carotid artery
26 Hypoglossus nerve (XII)
27 Atlas (anterior arch)
28 Vagus nerve (X)
29 Transverse process and foramen transversarium
30 Accessory nerve (XI)
31 Digastric muscle (posterior belly)
32 Atlas, lateral mass
33 Sternocleidomastoid muscle
34 Dens of axis
35 Spinal cord
36 Transverse ligament of atlas
37 Deep cervical veins
38 Longissimus capitis muscle
39 Trapezius muscle
40 Obliquus capitis inferior muscle
41 Semispinalis capitis muscle
42 Splenius capitis muscle
43 Nuchal ligament

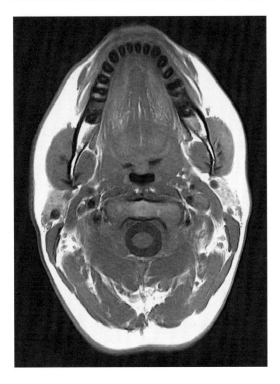

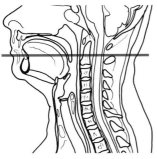

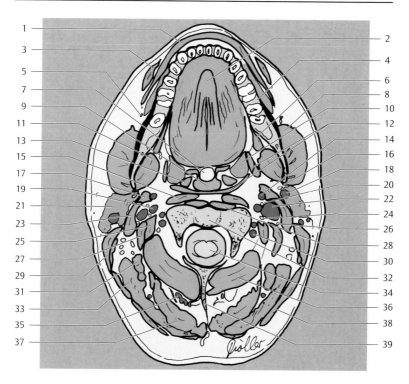

1 Orbicularis oris muscle
2 Tongue (genioglossus muscle)
3 Levator anguli oris muscle
4 Mandible
5 Facial artery
6 Hypoglossus muscle
7 Uvula
8 Masseter muscle
9 Oropharynx
10 Palatine tonsil
11 Medial pterygoid muscle
12 Superior constrictor muscle of pharynx
13 Palatopharyngeus muscle
14 External carotid artery
15 Longus capitis muscle
16 Facial nerve (VII)
17 Stylohyoid muscle, styloglossus muscle
18 Retromandibular vein
19 Internal carotid artery
20 Hypoglossus nerve (XII)
21 Parotid gland
22 Internal jugular vein
23 Digastric muscle (posterior belly)
24 Vagus nerve (X)
25 Longissimus cervicis muscle
26 Accessory nerve (XI)
27 Levator scapulae muscle
28 Longus colli muscle
29 Sternocleidomastoid muscle
30 Vertebral artery
31 Longissimus capitis muscle
32 Axis, body
33 Splenius capitis muscle
34 Spinal cord
35 Deep cervical veins
36 Obliquus capitis inferior muscle
37 Semispinalis capitis muscle
38 Trapezius muscle
39 Nuchal ligament

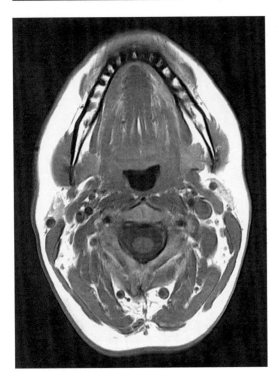

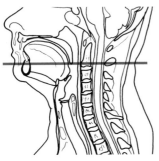

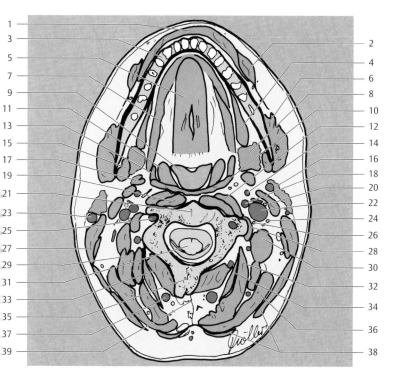

1 Orbicularis oris muscle
2 Depressor anguli oris muscle
3 Mandible
4 Mylohyoid muscle
5 Genioglossus muscle
6 Masseter muscle
7 Hyoglossus muscle
8 Submandibular gland
9 Oropharynx
10 Superior constrictor muscle of pharynx
11 Palatopharyngeus muscle
12 Longus capitis muscle
13 Middle constrictor muscle of pharynx
14 External carotid artery
15 Medial pterygoid muscle
16 Parotid gland
17 Styloglossus muscle and stylohyoid muscle
18 Internal carotid artery
19 Longus colli muscle
20 Hypoglossal nerve (XII)
21 Axis, body
22 Internal jugular vein
23 Retromandibular vein
24 Accessory nerve (XI)
25 Vertebral artery
26 Vagus nerve (X)
27 Sternocleidomastoid muscle
28 Longissimus cervicis muscle
29 Longissimus capitis muscle
30 Levator scapulae muscle
31 Spinal cord
32 Semispinalis capitis muscle
33 Spinalis capitis muscle and multifidus muscle
34 Semispinalis cervicis muscle
35 Spinous process of vertebra
36 Splenius capitis muscle
37 Deep cervical veins
38 Trapezius muscle
39 Nuchal ligament

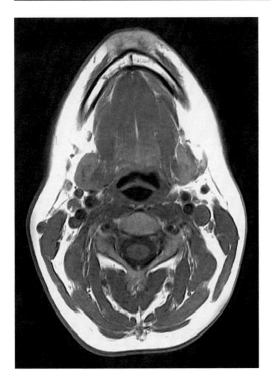

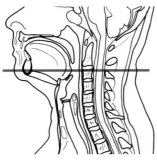

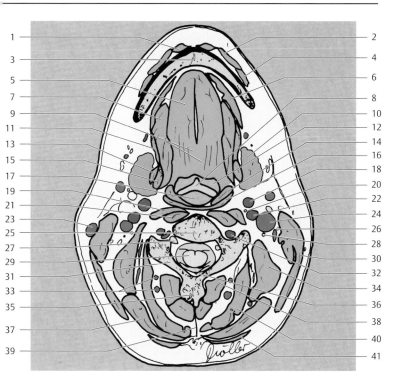

1 Mentalis muscle
2 Depressor anguli oris muscle
3 Mandible
4 Platysma
5 Genioglossus muscle
6 Mylohyoid muscle
7 Hyoglossus muscle
8 Epiglottis
9 Root of tongue
10 Submandibular gland
11 Styloglossus muscle
12 Oropharynx
13 Stylohyoid muscle
14 Palatopharyngeus muscle
15 Digastric muscle (posterior belly)
16 Middle constrictor muscle of pharynx
17 Hypopharynx
18 External carotid artery
19 Longus capitis muscle
20 Superior laryngeal nerve (vagus nerve)
21 Longus colli muscle
22 Internal carotid artery
23 External jugular vein
24 Internal jugular vein
25 Cervical vertebra C3 (body)
26 Accessory nerve (XI)
27 Spinal nerve root C4
28 Vagus nerve (X)
29 Spinal cord
30 Sternocleidomastoid muscle
31 Posterior arch of C3
32 Vertebral artery
33 Deep cervical veins
34 Levator scapulae muscle
35 Spinous process
36 Ligamentum flavum
37 Splenius capitis muscle
38 Spinalis cervicis muscle
39 Nuchal ligament
40 Semispinalis capitis muscle
41 Trapezius muscle

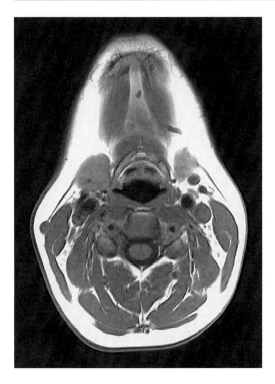

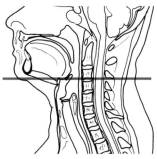

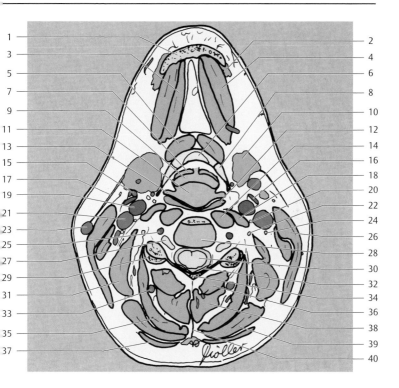

1 Mandible
2 Depressor anguli oris muscle
3 Mylohyoid muscle
4 Digastric muscle (anterior belly)
5 Geniohyoid muscle
6 Hyoid bone (body)
7 Epiglottic vallecula
8 Hyoid bone (greater horn)
9 Epiglottis
10 Submandibular gland
11 Hypopharynx
12 Inferior constrictor muscle of
    pharynx
13 Piriform recess
14 Longus colli muscle
15 Retromandibular vein
16 Superior thyroid artery
17 Platysma
18 Longus capitis muscle
19 Common carotid artery
    (bifurcation)
20 Vagus nerve (X)
21 Internal jugular vein
22 Spinal nerve (C3)
23 External jugular vein
24 Spinal nerve (C2)
25 Vertebral artery
26 Sternocleidomastoid muscle
27 Spinal nerve root (C4)
28 Intervertebral space (C3/C4)
29 Zygapophysial joint
30 Spinal cord
31 Levator scapulae muscle
32 Ligamentum flavum
33 Deep cervical veins
34 Posterior arch of C3 vertebra
35 Semispinalis capitis muscle
36 Spinalis cervicis muscle
37 Trapezius muscle
38 Semispinalis cervicis muscle
39 Splenius capitis muscle
40 Nuchal ligament

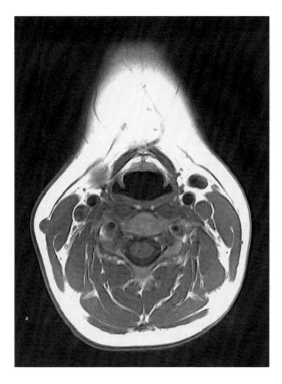

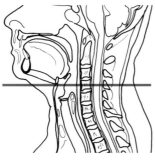

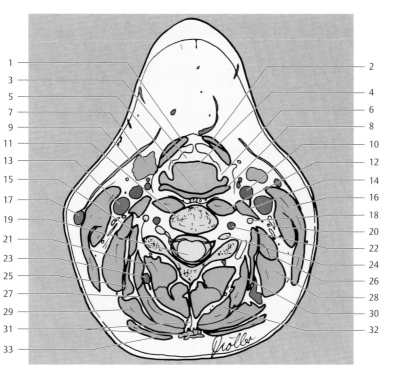

1 Thyrohyoid muscle
2 Sternohyoid muscle
3 Epiglottis (cartilage)
4 Laryngeal vestibule
5 Hypopharynx
6 Aryepiglottic fold
7 Submandibular gland
8 Inferior constrictor muscle of pharynx
9 Platysma
10 Common carotid artery
11 Cervical vertebra C4 (body)
12 Longus colli muscle
13 Internal jugular vein
14 Longus capitis muscle
15 Longissimus capitis muscle
16 Sternocleidomastoid muscle
17 External jugular vein
18 Spinal nerve (C4)
19 Spinal cord
20 Spinal nerve (C3)
21 Spinalis cervicis muscle
22 Vertebral artery
23 Deep cervical veins
24 Spinal nerve root (C5)
25 Longissimus cervicis muscle
26 Middle scalene muscle
27 Semispinalis cervicis muscle
28 Levator scapulae muscle
29 Splenius capitis muscle
30 Splenius cervicis muscle
31 Nuchal ligament
32 Semispinalis capitis muscle
33 Trapezius muscle

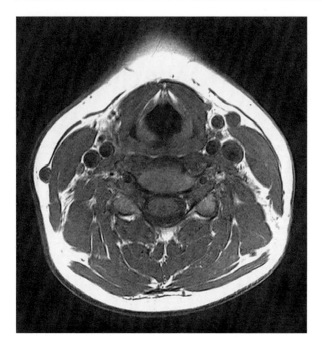

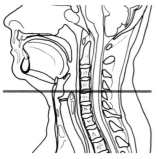

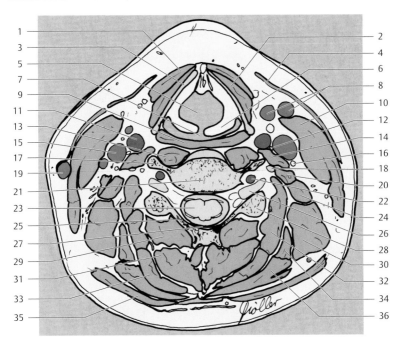

1 Sternohyoid muscle
2 Thyrohyoid muscle
3 Thyroid cartilage (lamina)
4 Platysma
5 Laryngeal vestibule
6 Aryepiglottic fold
7 Hypopharynx
8 Anterior jugular vein
9 Inferior constrictor muscle of
   pharynx
10 Sternocleidomastoid muscle
11 Common carotid artery
12 Vagus nerve (X)
13 Longus colli muscle
14 Longus capitis muscle
15 Internal jugular vein
16 Spinal nerve (C4)
17 Transverse process of C5
   vertebra
18 Spinal nerve (C5)
19 External jugular vein
20 Middle scalene muscle
21 Cervical vertebra C5 (body)
22 Vertebral artery
23 Spinal cord
24 Posterior scalene muscle
25 Posterior arch of C6 vertebra
26 Spinal nerve root (C6)
27 Ligamentum flavum
28 Inferior articular process
   of vertebra
29 Spinalis cervicis muscle and
   multifidus muscle
30 Levator scapulae muscle
31 Semispinalis cervicis muscle
32 Longissimus cervicis muscle
33 Semispinalis capitis muscle
34 Splenius cervicis muscle
35 Trapezius muscle
36 Splenius capitis muscle

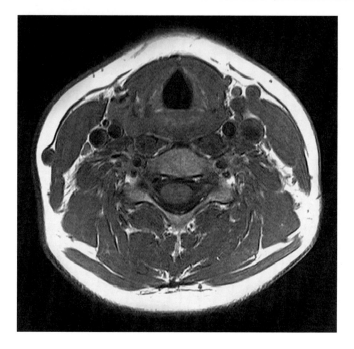

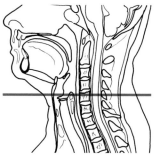

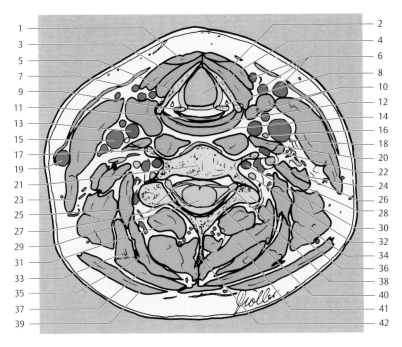

1 Sternohyoid muscle
2 Thyrohyoid muscle
3 Omohyoid muscle
4 Larynx
5 Thyroid cartilage (lamina)
6 Anterior jugular vein
7 Platysma
8 Piriform recess
9 Arytenoid cartilage
10 Thyroid gland
11 Cricoid cartilage
12 Hypopharynx
13 Common carotid artery
14 Inferior constrictor muscle of
   pharynx
15 Internal jugular vein
16 Vagus nerve (X)
17 Longus colli muscle
18 Phrenic nerve
19 External jugular vein
20 Longus capitis muscle
21 Cervical vertebra C5 (body)

22 Anterior scalene muscle
23 Sternocleidomastoid muscle
24 Posterior scalene muscle
25 Longissimus cervicis muscle
26 Spinal nerve (C4)
27 Anterior and posterior nerve roots
28 Middle scalene muscle
29 Spinal cord
30 Vertebral artery
31 Spinalis cervicis muscle and
   multifidus muscle
32 Spinal nerve (C5)
33 Splenius cervicis muscle
34 Levator scapulae muscle
35 Semispinalis capitis muscle
36 Inferior articular process of vertebra
37 Splenius capitis nerve
38 Spinal nerve root (C6)
39 Trapezius muscle
40 Posterior arch of C6 vertebra
41 Semispinalis cervicis muscle
42 Spinous process of C6 vertebra

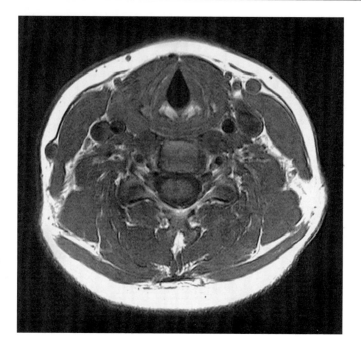

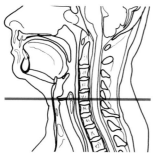

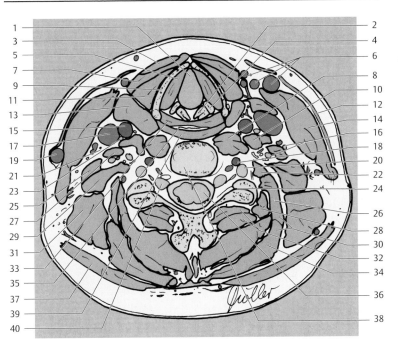

1 Glottis
2 Cricoid cartilage
3 Sternohyoid muscle
4 Arytenoid cartilage
5 Vocalis muscle
6 Anterior jugular vein
7 Omohyoid muscle
8 Longus colli muscle
9 Thyroid cartilage (lamina)
10 Longus capitis muscle
11 Thyrohyoid muscle
12 Platysma
13 Thyroid gland
14 Sternocleidomastoid muscle
15 Common carotid artery
16 Spinal nerves (C4 and C5)
17 Internal jugular vein
18 Vertebral artery
19 External jugular vein
20 Spinal nerve (C6)
21 Phrenic nerve
22 Longissimus capitis muscle
23 Vagus nerve (X)
24 Zygapophysial joint
25 Middle scalene muscle
26 Longissimus cervicis muscle
27 Anterior scalene muscle
28 Semispinalis capitis muscle
29 Posterior scalene muscle
30 Splenius cervicis muscle and splenius capitis muscle
31 Levator scapulae muscle
32 Spinalis cervicis muscle and multifidus muscle
33 Posterior cricoarytenoid muscle
34 Semispinalis cervicis muscle
35 Hypopharynx/esophagus
36 Spinal cord
37 Trapezius muscle
38 Cervical vertebra C5
39 Inferior constrictor muscle of pharynx
40 Nerve root (C7)

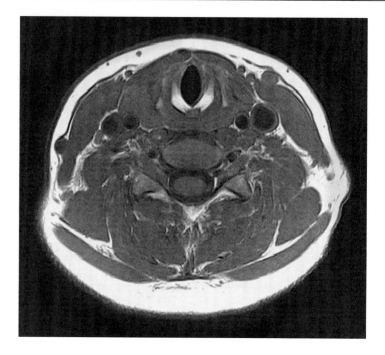

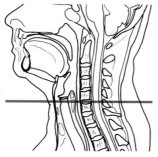

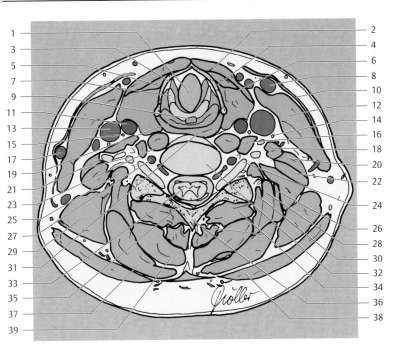

1 Larynx
2 Sternohyoid muscle
3 Vocalis muscle (vocal cord)
4 Thyroid cartilage (lamina)
5 Thyrohyoid muscle
6 Thyroid gland
7 Arytenoid cartilage
8 Anterior jugular vein
9 Transverse arytenoid muscle
10 Platysma
11 Common carotid artery
12 Sternocleidomastoid muscle
13 Internal jugular vein
14 Phrenic muscle
15 Vagus nerve (X)
16 Longus capitis muscle
17 External jugular vein
18 Anterior scalene muscle
19 Hypopharynx/esophagus
20 Middle scalene muscle
21 Spinal nerves (C4 and C5)
22 Posterior scalene muscle
23 Longus colli muscle
24 Spinal nerve root (C6)
25 Longissimus capitis muscle
26 Longissimus cervicis muscle
27 Vertebral artery
28 Splenius cervicis muscle
29 Levator scapulae muscle
30 Semispinalis capitis muscle
31 Inferior constrictor muscle of pharynx
32 Intervertebral space (C5/C6)
33 Spinal cord
34 Spinalis cervicis muscle and multifidus muscle
35 Ligamentum flavum
36 Posterior vertebral arch
37 Splenius capitis muscle
38 Trapezius muscle
39 Semispinalis cervicis muscle

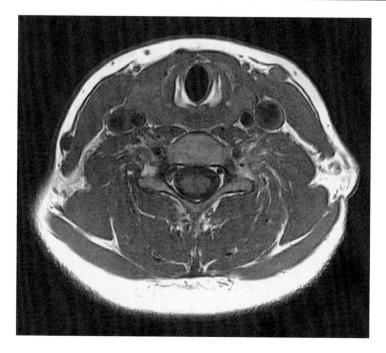

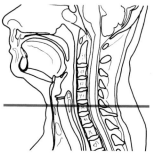

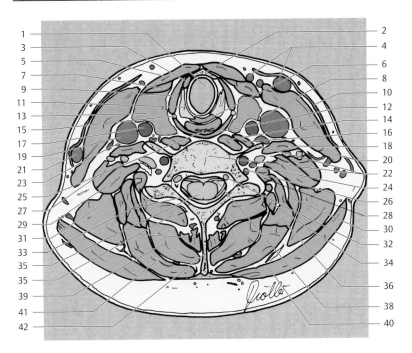

1 Larynx
3 Thyro-arytenoid muscle
5 Sternohyoid muscle
7 Thyrohyoid muscle
9 Sternothyroid muscle
11 Cricoid cartilage (lamina)
13 Thyroid gland
15 Thyroid cartilage (inferior horn)
17 Common carotid artery
19 Internal jugular vein
21 External jugular vein

2 Thyroid cartilage
4 Anterior jugular vein
6 Transverse arytenoid muscle
8 Vagus nerve (X)
10 Platysma
12 Inferior constrictor muscle of pharynx
14 Longus colli muscle
16 Longus capitis muscle
18 Anterior scalene muscle
20 Sternocleidomastoid muscle
22 Cervical vertebra (C6)

1 Larynx
2 Thyroid cartilage
3 Thyro-arytenoid muscle
4 Anterior jugular vein
5 Sternohyoid muscle
6 Transverse arytenoid muscle
7 Thyrohyoid muscle
8 Vagus nerve (X)
9 Sternothyroid muscle
10 Platysma
11 Cricoid cartilage (lamina)
12 Inferior constrictor muscle of pharynx
13 Thyroid gland
14 Longus colli muscle
15 Thyroid cartilage (inferior horn)
16 Longus capitis muscle
17 Common carotid artery
18 Anterior scalene muscle
19 Internal jugular vein
20 Sternocleidomastoid muscle
21 External jugular vein
22 Cervical vertebra (C6)
23 Phrenic nerve
24 Spinal nerves (C4, C5, and C6)
25 Esophagus
26 Vertebral artery
27 Middle scalene muscle
28 Longissimus capitis muscle
29 Posterior scalene muscle
30 Longissimus cervicis muscle
31 Levator scapulae muscle
32 Spinal nerve root (C7)
33 Articular process and posterior arch of C7 vertebra
34 Semispinalis capitis muscle
35 Spinal cord
36 Splenius cervicis muscle
37 Spinalis cervicis muscle and multifidus muscle
38 Anterior and posterior spinal nerve roots (C8)
39 Semispinalis cervicis muscle
40 Trapezius muscle
41 Splenius capitis muscle
42 Spinous process of vertebra

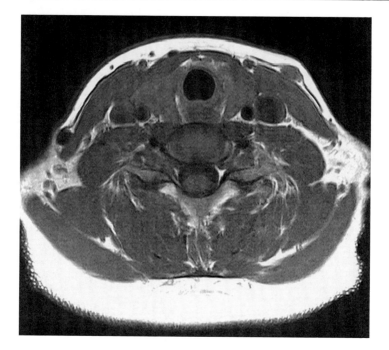

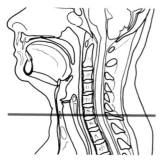

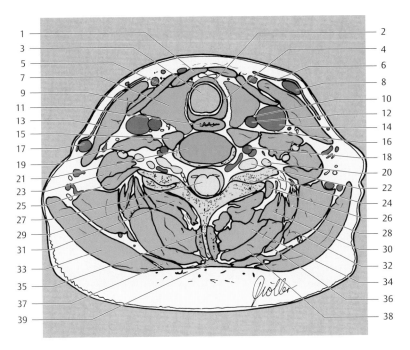

1 Sternohyoid muscle
2 Cricoid cartilage (arch)
3 Trachea
4 Cricothyroid muscle
5 Sternothyroid muscle
6 Platysma
7 Thyroid gland
8 Anterior jugular vein
9 Omohyoid muscle
10 Vagus nerve (X)
11 Esophagus
12 Common carotid artery
13 Sternocleidomastoid muscle
14 Internal jugular vein
15 Longus colli muscle
16 Phrenic muscle
17 External jugular vein
18 Vertebral artery
19 Anterior scalene muscle
20 Spinal nerves (C4, C5, and C6)
21 Intervertebral space (C6/C7)
22 Spinal nerve root (C7)
23 Middle scalene muscle
24 Zygapophysial joint (C6/C7)
25 Posterior scalene muscle
26 Longissimus capitis muscle
27 Spinal cord
28 Longissimus cervicis muscle
29 Semispinalis capitis muscle
30 Splenius cervicis muscle
31 Spinalis cervicis muscle and multifidus muscle
32 Levator scapulae muscle
33 Trapezius muscle
34 Semispinalis cervicis muscle
35 Spinous process of vertebra
36 Serratus posterior superior muscle
37 Rhomboid minor muscle
38 Splenius capitis muscle
39 Nuchal ligament

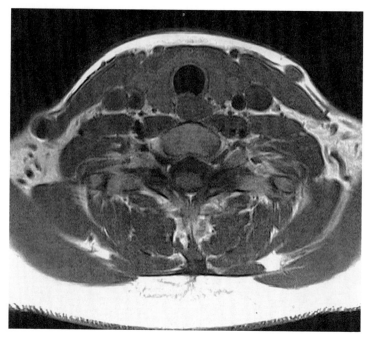

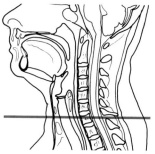

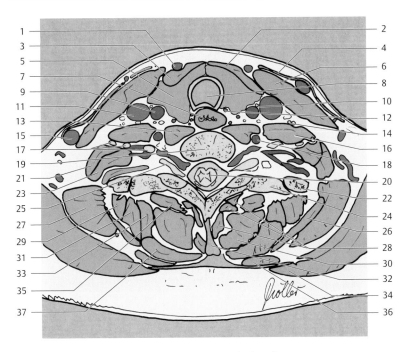

1 Anterior jugular vein
2 Sternohyoid muscle
3 Sternothyoid muscle
4 Platysma
5 Thyroid gland
6 Sternocleidomastoid muscle
7 Esophagus
8 Trachea
9 Common carotid artery
10 Vagus nerve (X)
11 Internal jugular vein
12 Inferior thyroid artery
13 Longus colli muscle
14 Phrenic nerve
15 External jugular vein
16 Anterior scalene muscle
17 Spinal nerves (C5, C6, and C7)
18 Vertebral artery
19 Cervical vertebra (C7)
20 Spinal cord
21 Middle scalene muscle
22 First rib
23 Posterior scalene muscle
24 Transverse process of vertebra
25 Spinal nerve root (C8)
26 Serratus posterior superior muscle
27 Levator scapulae muscle
28 Spinalis cervicis muscle and multifidus muscle
29 Iliocostalis cervicis muscle
30 Semispinalis cervicis muscle
31 Longissimus cervicis muscle
32 Interspinous ligament
33 Splenius cervicis muscle
34 Trapezius muscle
35 Semispinalis capitis muscle
36 Rhomboid minor muscle
37 Splenius capitis muscle

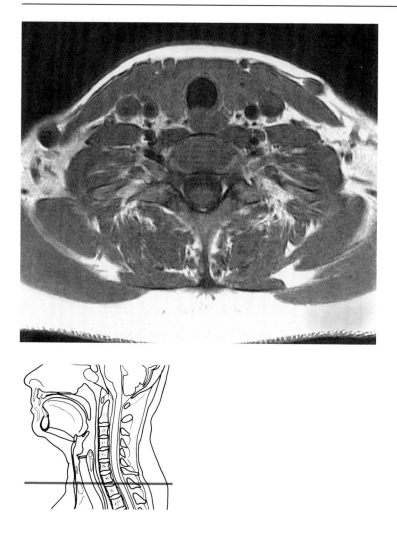

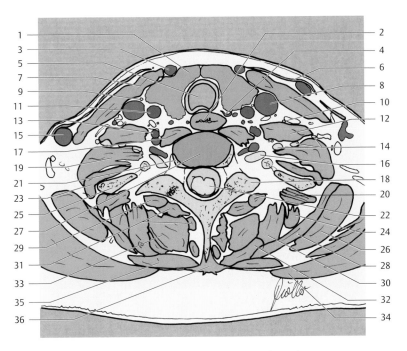

1 Thyroid gland
2 Esophagus
3 Anterior jugular vein
4 Inferior thyroid vein
5 Trachea
6 Platysma
7 Sternocleidomastoid muscle
8 Internal jugular vein
9 Vagus nerve (X)
10 Phrenic nerve
11 Common carotid artery
12 Anterior scalene muscle
13 Vertebral artery
14 Spinal nerves (C5, C6, and C7)
15 External jugular vein
16 Spinal nerve root (C8)
17 Longus colli muscle
18 Transverse process of T1 vertebra
19 Middle scalene muscle
20 Intercostal muscles
21 Superior posterior margin of T1 vertebra
22 Spinal cord
23 Posterior scalene muscle
24 Iliocostalis cervicis muscle
25 First rib
26 Levator scapulae muscle
27 Intervertebral space (C7/T1)
28 Serratus posterior superior muscle
29 Semispinalis capitis muscle
30 Splenius cervicis muscle
31 Spinalis cervicis muscle and multifidus muscle
32 Splenius capitis muscle
33 Semispinalis cervicis muscle
34 Trapezius muscle
35 Rhomboid minor muscle
36 Interspinous ligament

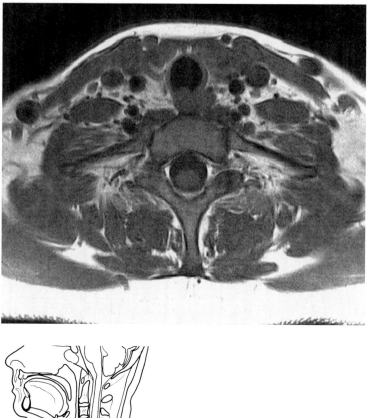

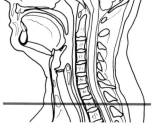

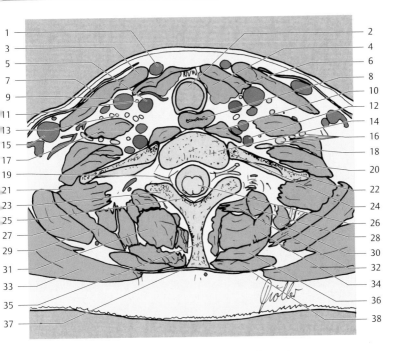

1 Anterior jugular vein
2 Trachea
3 Sternocleidomastoid muscle
4 Thyroid gland
5 Common carotid artery
6 Sternohyoid muscle
7 Platysma
8 Esophagus
9 Internal jugular vein
10 Longus colli muscle
11 Vagus nerve (X)
12 Vertebral artery
13 Phrenic nerve
14 Vertebra (T1)
15 External jugular vein
16 Cervical plexus (C5 to C8)
17 Anterior scalene muscle
18 Middle scalene muscle
19 Spinal nerve root (T1)
20 Posterior scalene muscle

21 Intercostal muscles
22 First rib
23 Transverse process of T1 vertebra
24 Costovertebral joint
25 Ligamentum flavum
26 Spinal cord
27 Levator scapulae muscle
28 Semispinalis capitis muscle
29 Serratus posterior superior muscle
30 Iliocostalis cervicis muscle
31 Semispinalis cervicis muscle
32 Spinalis cervicis muscle and
multifidus muscle
33 Trapezius muscle
34 Splenius cervicis muscle
35 Spinous process of vertebra
36 Splenius capitis muscle
37 Interspinous ligament
38 Rhomboid minor muscle

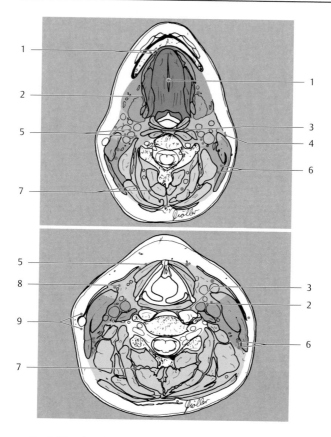

Cervical lymph nodes

1 Submental lymph nodes
2 Submandibular lymph nodes
3 Retropharyngeal lymph nodes
4 Preauricular lymph nodes
5 Superior jugular group of lymph nodes
6 Deep cervical lymph nodes
7 Nuchal lymph nodes
8 Anterior jugular lymph nodes
9 Superficial cervical lymph nodes

Lymph nodes (classified according to levels)

Level 1a (submental lymph nodes between digastric muscles)

Level 1b (submandibular lymph nodes)

Level 2a (lymph nodes anterior, medial, or lateral to the internal jugular vein)

Level 2b (Lymph nodes dorsal to the internal jugular vein and separated from the vein by a lamella of fat)

Level 3 (lymph nodes along the jugular vein)

Level 5a (lymph nodes in the posterior triangle, upper level = above arch of cricoid cartilage)

Level 6 (upper visceral lymph nodes: ventral between the carotid arteries)

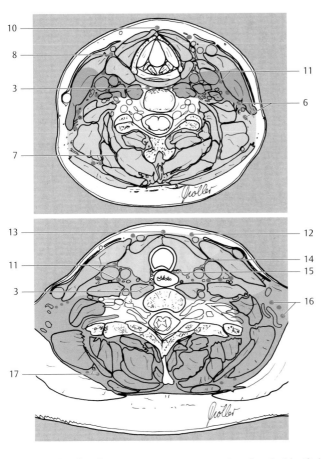

Cervical lymph nodes

3 Retropharyngeal lymph nodes
6 Deep cervical lymph nodes
7 Nuchal lymph nodes
8 Anterior jugular lymph nodes
10 Prelaryngeal lymph nodes
11 Inferior jugular group of lymph nodes
12 Anterior cervical lymph nodes
13 Pretracheal lymph nodes
14 Thyroid lymph nodes
15 Paratracheal lymph nodes
16 Supraclavicular lymph nodes
17 Superficial cervical lymph nodes

Lymph nodes (classified according to levels)

Level 3 (lymph nodes along the jugular vein)

Level 4 (lymph nodes of the lower jugular vein)

Level 5a (lymph nodes of the posterior triangle, upper level = above arch of cricoid cartilage)

Level 5b (lymph nodes of the posterior triangle, lower level = below arch of cricoid cartilage)

Level 6 (upper visceral lymph nodes: ventral between the carotid arteries)

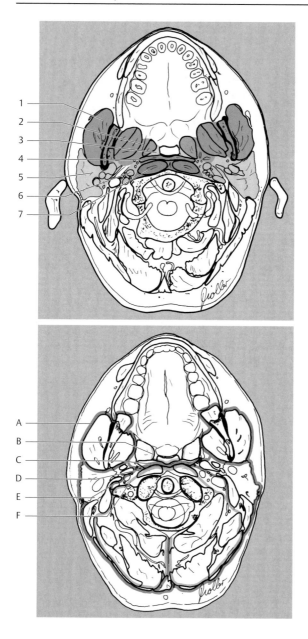

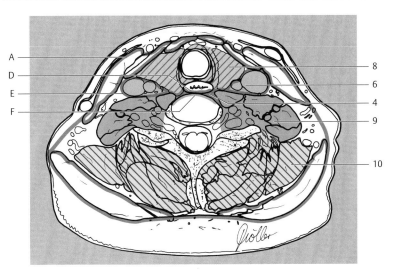

Müller

Cervical spaces

1 Masticatory space (chewing muscles, ramus and body of mandible, inferior alveolar nerve, maxillary artery, pterygoid plexus, lingual nerve)

2 Parapharyngeal space (trigeminal nerve, pharyngeal artery)

3 Superficial mucosal space (submucosal salivary glands, lymphatic tissue)

4 Retropharyngeal space

5 Parotid space (parotid gland, facial nerve, external carotid artery, retromandibular vein)

6 Carotid space (carotid artery, jugular vein, cranial nerves IX–XII, sympathetic trunk)

7 Prevertebral space (prevertebral and paraspinal muscles, phrenic nerve)

8 Visceral space (thyroid gland, paratracheal space)

9 Perivertebral space (prevertebral part)

10 Perivertebral space (paraspinal part)

Cervical fasciae

A Superficial cervical fascia (fascia colli superficialis)

B Pharyngobasilar fascia

C Middle layer of deep cervical fascia (pretracheal layer)

D Intercarotid fascia

E Carotid sheath

F Deep layer of deep cervical fascia (prevertebral layer)

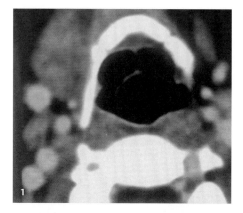

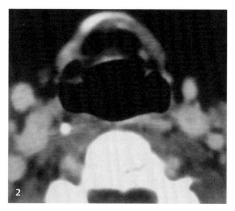

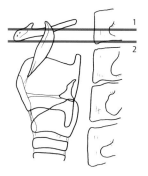

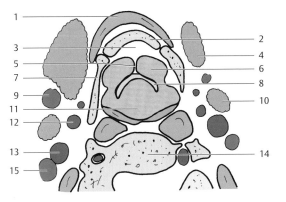

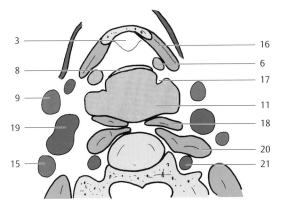

1 Suprahyoid muscles (mylo-
   and geniohyoid muscles,
   hypoglossus muscle)
2 Hyoid bone (body)
3 Pre-epiglottic space
4 Submandibular gland
5 Glossoepiglottic fold
6 Epiglottic vallecula
7 Hyoid bone (greater horn)
8 Epiglottis
9 Anterior jugular vein
10 Parotid gland
11 Hypopharynx
12 External carotid artery
13 Internal carotid artery
14 Cervical vertebra (C3)
15 Internal jugular vein
16 Infrahyoid muscles (sternohyoid
   and sternothyroid muscles)
17 Pharyngoepiglottic fold
18 Inferior constrictor muscle of
   pharynx
19 Carotid bifurcation
20 Longus colli muscle
21 Vertebral artery

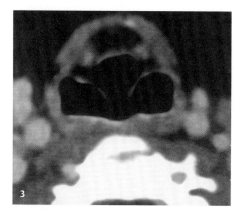

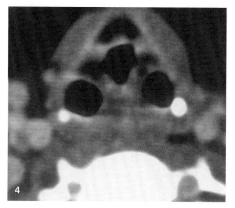

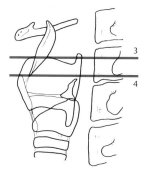

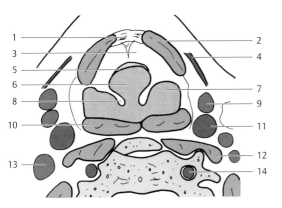

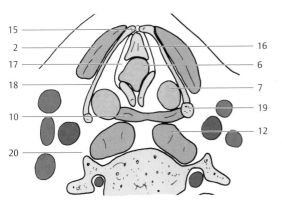

1 Thyrohyoid membrane
2 Infrahyoid muscles
  (sternothyroid, omohyoid,
  thyrohyoid)
3 Pre-epiglottic space
4 Platysma
5 Epiglottis
6 Larynx
7 Piriform recess
8 Aryepiglottic fold
9 Anterior jugular vein

10 Inferior constrictor muscle of pharynx
11 Common carotid artery
12 Longus colli muscle
13 Internal jugular vein
14 Vertebral artery
15 Superior thyroid notch
16 Stalk of epiglottis
17 Vestibular folds
18 Thyroid cartilage (lamina)
19 Thyroid cartilage (superior horn)
20 Body of cervical vertebra (C4)

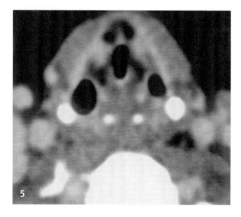

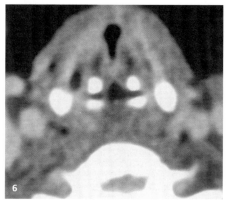

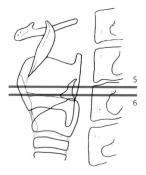

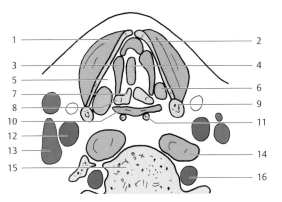

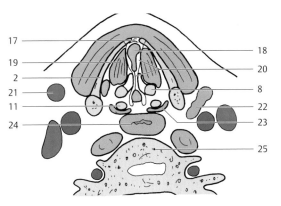

1 Infrahyoid muscles
   (sternothyroid, omohyoid and
   thyrohyoid muscles)
2 Thyroid cartilage
3 Thyro-arytenoid muscle
4 Larynx (vestibule)
5 Paralaryngeal space
6 Piriform recess
7 Arytenoid cartilage (vocal
   process)
8 Arytenoid cartilage (body)
9 Thyroid cartilage
   (superior horn)
10 Transverse arytenoid muscle
11 Cricoid cartilage

12 Common carotid artery
13 Internal jugular vein
14 Longus colli muscle
15 Body of cervical vertebra C4
16 Vertebral artery
17 Laryngeal prominence
18 Rima glottidis
19 Vocalis muscle
20 True vocal cord
21 Anterior jugular vein
22 Thyroid gland
23 Oblique arytenoid muscle
24 Esophagus
25 Body of cervical vertebra C5

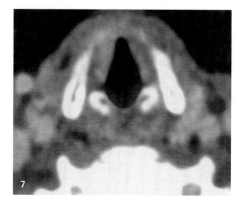

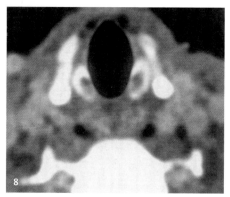

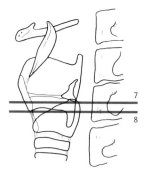

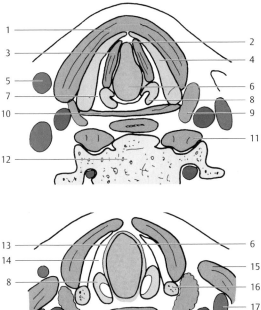

1 Infrahyoid muscles (sternohyoid, omohyoid and sternothyroid muscles)
2 Anterior laryngeal commissure
3 Vocalis muscle
4 Thyroid cartilage
5 Anterior jugular vein
6 Infraglottic cavity
7 Cricothyroid joint
8 Cricoid cartilage (lamina)
9 Thyroid gland
10 Inferior constrictor muscle of pharynx
11 Longus colli muscle
12 Body of cervical vertebra (C6)
13 Conus elasticus (cricovocal membrane)
14 Paralaryngeal space
15 Sternocleidomastoid muscle
16 Thyroid cartilage (inferior horn)
17 Internal jugular vein
18 Common carotid artery
19 Esophagus
20 Vertebral artery

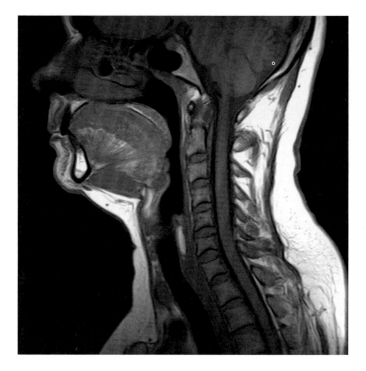

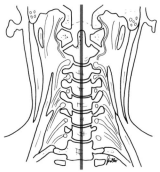

1	Palatine tonsil	6	Apical ligament of dens
2	Foramen magnum	7	Hard palate
3	Vomer	8	Tectorial membrane
4	Anterior longitudinal ligament	9	Incisive canal
5	Nasopharynx and longus colli muscle	10	Posterior atlanto-occipital membrane
		11	Orbicularis oris muscle

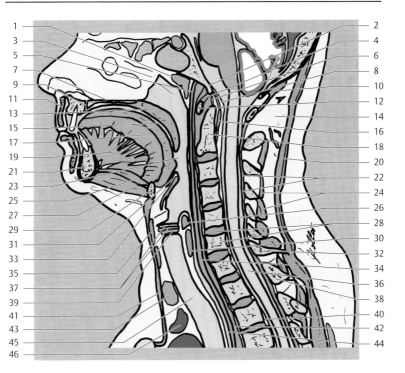

12 Anterior arch of atlas
13 Soft palate
14 Suboccipital fatty tissue
15 Superior longitudinal muscle
    of tongue and oral cavity
16 Transverse ligament of atlas
    (of cruciform ligament
    of atlas)
17 Transverse muscle of tongue
18 Dens of axis (C2)
19 Genioglossus muscle and
    lingual septum
20 Nuchal ligament
21 Mandible
22 Ligamentum flavum
23 Oropharynx
24 Interspinalis muscles
25 Geniohyoid muscle
26 Transverse and oblique
    arytenoid muscles
27 Mylohyoid muscle

28 Vertebra C6 and intervertebral disc
29 Hyoid bone
30 Larynx (lamina)
31 Epiglottis
32 Spinous process of C7
33 Epiglottic vallecula
34 Inferior constrictor muscle of
    pharynx
35 Thyroid cartilage
36 Spinal cord
37 Vestibular ligament and laryngeal
    ventricle (ventricle of Morgagni)
38 Spinous process
39 Vocal ligament (false vocal cord)
40 Posterior longitudinal ligament
41 Sternothyroid muscle
42 Anterior longitudinal ligament
43 Thyroid gland
44 Esophagus
45 Trachea
46 Brachiocephalic artery

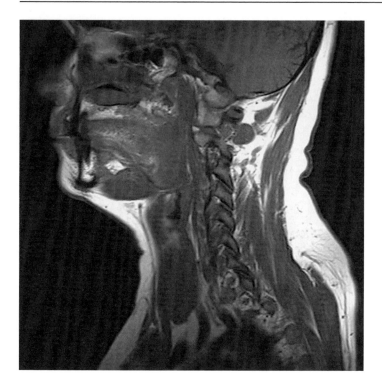

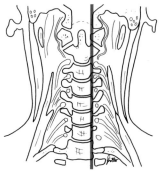

1 Levator veli palatini muscle
2 Semispinalis capitis muscle
3 Medial pterygoid muscle
4 Atlas (lateral mass)

5 Longus capitis muscle
6 Rectus capitis posterior minor muscle
7 Maxilla
8 Rectus capitis posterior major muscle

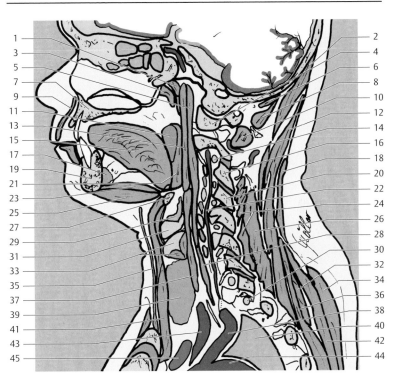

9 Orbicularis oris muscle
10 Inferior oblique muscle
11 Palatine tonsil
12 Splenius capitis muscle
13 Superior constrictor muscle of pharynx
14 Spinal nerve root (C3)
15 Tongue
16 Inferior articular process
17 Sublingual gland
18 Trapezius muscle (descending part)
19 Mandible
20 Superior articular process
21 Palatopharyngeus muscle
22 Vertebral artery
23 Mylohoid muscle
24 Multifidus muscle
25 Digastric muscle (anterior belly)
26 Semispinalis cervicis muscle
27 Hyoid bone
28 Longus colli muscle
29 Pharynx and epiglottic vallecula
30 Spinal nerve root (T1)
31 Thyroid cartilage
32 Serratus posterior superior muscle
33 Cricoid cartilage
34 Trapezius muscle
35 Platysma
36 Splenius cervicis muscle
37 Inferior constrictor muscle of pharynx
38 Left subclavian artery
39 Thyroid gland
40 Left lung
41 Sternohyoid muscle
42 Rhomboid (major and minor) muscle
43 Common carotid artery
44 Aortic arch
45 Left brachiocephalic vein

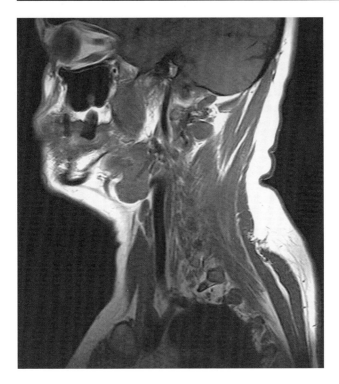

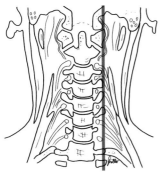

1 Maxillary sinus
2 Internal carotid artery (carotid syphon)
3 Medial pterygoid muscle
4 Mandibular nerve
5 Levator labii superioris muscle
6 Pharyngotympanic tube (auditory tube)
7 Digastric muscle

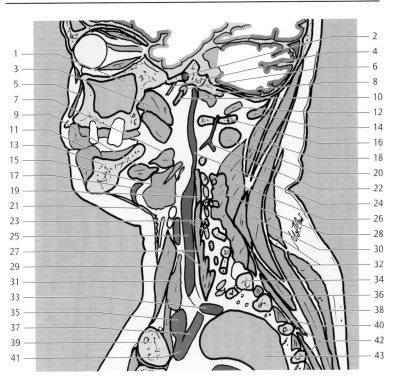

8 Rectus capitis lateralis muscle
9 Mylohyoid muscle
10 Tensor veli palatini muscle
11 Orbicularis orbis muscle
12 Obliquus capitis superior muscle
13 Mandible
14 Rectus capitis posterior major muscle
15 Submandibular gland
16 Atlas (transverse process)
17 Facial vein
18 Semispinalis capitis muscle
19 Longus colli muscle
20 Obliquus capitis inferior muscle
21 Platysma
22 Vertebral artery
23 Transverse processes and spinal nerve roots
24 Internal carotid artery

25 Common carotid artery
26 Semispinalis cervicis muscle
27 Scalenus anterior muscle
28 Scalenus posterior muscle
29 Sternocleidomastoid muscle
30 Splenius capitis muscle
31 Thyroid gland
32 Trapezius muscle
33 Subclavian artery
34 First rib
35 Internal jugular vein
36 Semispinalis cervicis muscle
37 Subclavian vein (left)
38 Rhomboid (major and minor) muscle
39 Clavicle
40 Interspinalis muscle
41 Brachiocephalic vein (left)
42 Serratus anterior muscle
43 Lung (left)

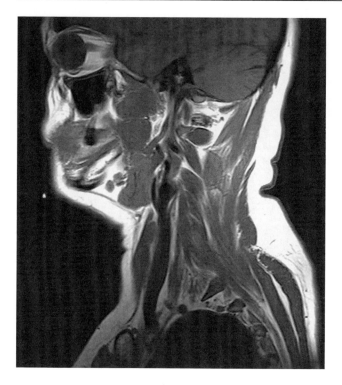

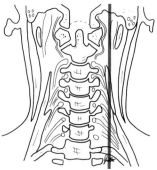

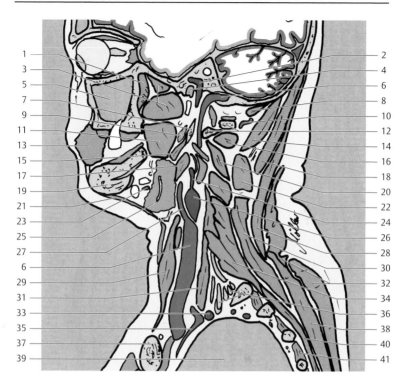

1 Temporal muscle
2 Internal carotid artery (syphon)
3 Lateral pterygoid muscle
4 Pharyngotympanic tube (auditory tube)
5 Maxillary sinus
6 Internal jugular vein
7 Styloid process
8 Rectus capitis posterior minor muscle
9 Parotid gland
10 Deep cervical veins
11 Medial pterygoid muscle
12 Atlas (transverse process)
13 Buccinator muscle
14 Rectus capitis posterior major muscle
15 Stylohyoid muscle
16 Obliquus capitis muscle
17 Digastric muscle
18 Semispinalis capitis muscle
19 Mandible
20 Levator scapulae muscle
21 Platysma
22 Semispinalis cervicis muscle
23 Facial vein
24 External carotid artery
25 Submandibular gland
26 Common carotid artery
27 External jugular vein
28 Splenius capitis muscle
29 Sternocleidomastoid muscle
30 Semispinalis cervicis muscle
31 Scalenus medius muscle
32 Trapezius muscle
33 Subclavian artery (left)
34 Scalenus posterior muscle
35 Subclavian vein (left)
36 Brachial plexus
37 Clavicle
38 Rhomboid (major and minor) muscle
39 Lung (left)
40 Multifidus muscle
41 Interspinalis muscle

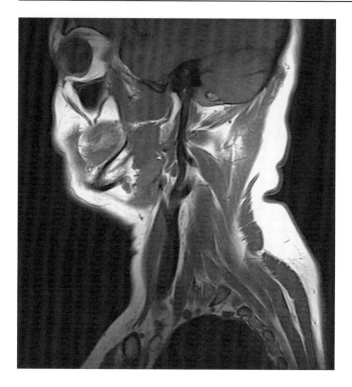

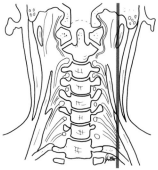

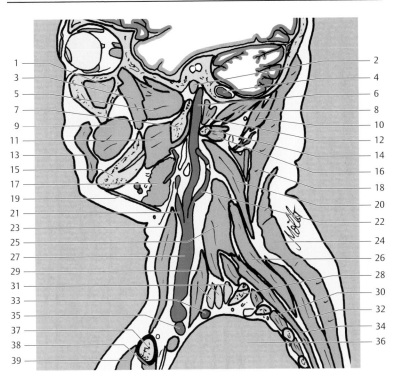

1 Maxillary sinus
2 External acoustic meatus
3 Temporal muscle
4 Sigmoid sinus
5 Lateral pterygoid muscle
6 Internal jugular vein
7 Ramus of the mandible
8 Obliquus capitis posterior major and minor muscles
9 Buccinator muscle
10 Semispinalis capitis muscle
11 Medial pterygoid muscle
12 Rectus capitis lateralis muscle
13 Orbicularis oris muscle
14 Transverse process of cervical vertebra C1
15 Mandible
16 Obliquus capitis superior muscle
17 Submandibular gland
18 Splenius capitis muscle
19 Platysma
20 Levator scapulae muscle
21 Common facial vein
22 Cervical veins
23 Sternocleidomastoid muscle
24 Trapezius muscle
25 Scalenus medius muscle
26 Semispinalis cervicis muscle
27 Internal jugular vein
28 First rib
29 Scalenus anterior muscle
30 Interspinalis muscle
31 Brachial plexus
32 Rhomboid (major and minor) muscle
33 Subclavian artery (left)
34 Serratus anterior muscle
35 Subclavian vein (left)
36 Lung
37 Clavicle
38 Subclavian muscle
39 Pectoralis major muscle

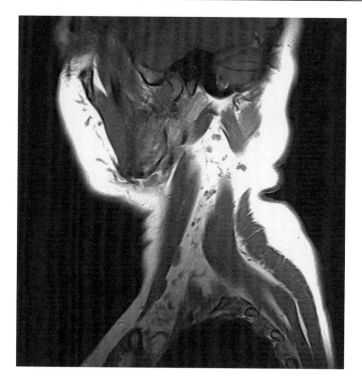

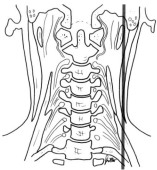

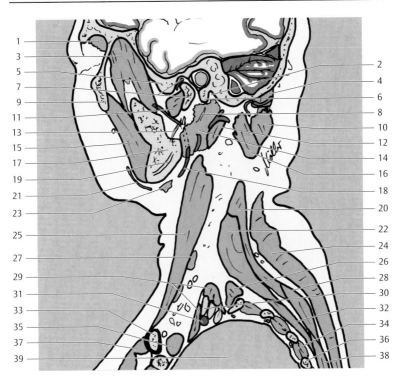

1 Lacrimal gland
2 Stylomastoid foramen
3 Temporal muscle
4 Obliquus capitis superior muscle
5 Articular tubercle
6 Styloid process
7 Head of mandible and articular disc
8 Facial nerve
9 Zygomatic bone
10 Splenius capitis muscle
11 Lateral pterygoid muscle
12 Digastric muscle (posterior belly)
13 Inferior alveolar nerve
14 Parotid gland
15 Masseter muscle
16 Semispinalis capitis muscle
17 Mandible
18 External carotid artery
19 Mandibular canal
20 Levator scapulae muscle
21 Platysma
22 Scalenus posterior muscle
23 Submandibular gland
24 Trapezius muscle
25 Sternocleidomastoid muscle
26 Scalenus medius muscle
27 Lymph nodes
28 Rhomboid minor muscle
29 Scalenus anterior muscle
30 Brachial plexus
31 Subclavian artery (left)
32 Serratus anterior muscle
33 Clavicle
34 Interspinalis muscle
35 Subclavian muscle
36 Fourth rib
37 Pectoralis major muscle
38 Rhomboid major muscle
39 Lung (left)

Nasal vestibule
(nasal cavity)

Nasopharynx

Oral cavity proper

Isthmus of fauces (oropharyngeal isthmus)

Oropharynx

Laryngeal part of pharynx

Esophagus

Laryngeal vestibule

Laryngeal ventricle

Infraglottic cavity

Trachea

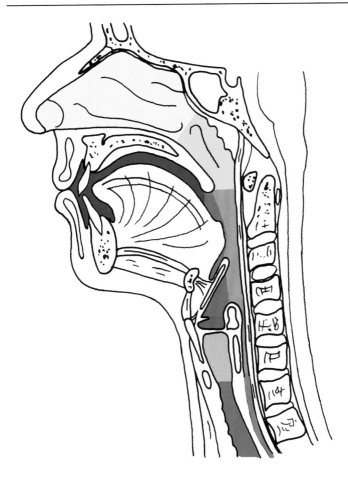

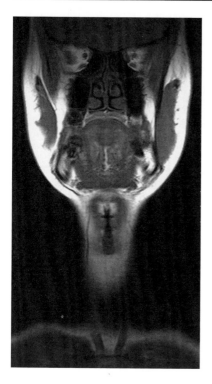

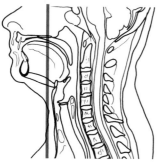

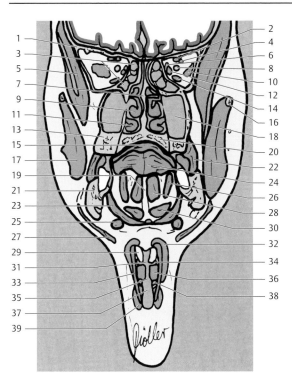

1 Sphenoidal bone (lesser wing)
2 Levator palpebrae superioris
   muscle
3 Ethmoidal cells (anterior)
4 Superior rectus muscle
5 Temporal muscle
6 Superior oblique muscle
7 Nasal septum
8 Optic nerve (II)
9 Middle nasal concha
10 Lateral rectus muscle
11 Inferior nasal concha
12 Medial rectus muscle
13 Mandible
14 Inferior rectus muscle
15 Longitudinal muscle of tongue
16 Zygomatic bone (temporal
   process)
17 Masseter muscle
18 Maxillary sinus
19 Lingual septum

20 Hard palate
21 Mandible
22 Buccinator muscle
23 Mylohoid muscle
24 Transverse muscle of tongue
25 Digastric muscle (anterior belly)
26 Hypoglossus muscle
27 Platysma
28 Genioglossus muscle
29 Vestibular fold
30 Geniohyoid muscle
31 Glottis
32 Thyrohyoid muscle
33 Thyroid cartilage
34 Laryngeal ventricle
35 Infraglottic cavity
36 Vocalis muscle
37 Trachea
38 Cricoid cartilage
39 Sternohyoid muscle

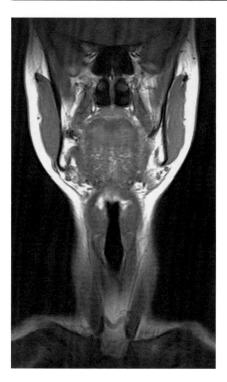

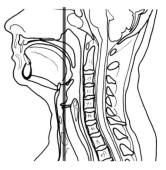

1 Superior orbital fissure
2 Optic nerve (II)
3 Sphenoidal bone (lesser wing)
4 Trochlear nerve (IV)

5 Temporal bone
6 Frontal nerve
7 Foramen rotundum with maxillary nerve (V2)

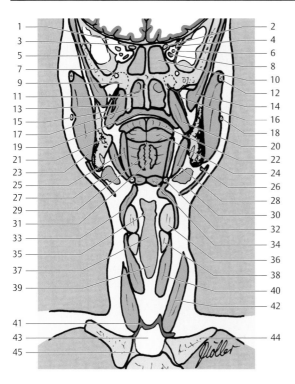

8 Superior ophthalmic vein
9 Pterygopalatine fossa
10 Sphenoidal sinus
11 Dorsal nasal cavity and nasal
    septum
12 Zygomatic bone (temporal
    process)
13 Pterygoid fossa
14 Temporal muscle
15 Lateral pterygoid process
16 Maxillary artery
17 Medial pterygoid process
18 Facial nerve (VII)
19 Soft palate
20 Medial pterygoid muscle
21 Mandible (ramus)
22 Longitudinal muscle of tongue
23 Masseter muscle
24 Transverse muscle of tongue
25 Hypoglossus muscle

26 Facial artery
27 Submandibular gland
28 Mylohoid muscle
29 Vertical muscle of tongue
30 Platysma
31 Lingual septum
32 Hyoid bone
33 Thyrohyoid muscle
34 Geniohyoid muscle
35 Laryngeal ventricle
36 Thyroid cartilage
37 Infraglottic cavity
38 Cricoid cartilage
39 Larynx
40 Cricothyroid muscle
41 Anterior jugular vein
42 Sternohyoid muscle
43 Suprasternal space
44 Clavicle
45 Sternoclavicular joint

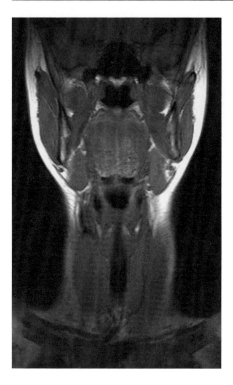

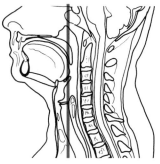

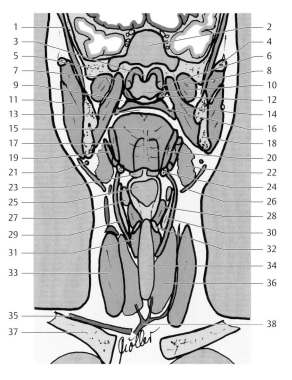

1 Temporal muscle
2 Sphenoidal sinus
3 Vomer
4 Zygomatic bone (temporal process)
5 Sphenoidal bone (greater wing)
6 Pharyngotympanic tube (auditory tube) (cartilage)
7 Lateral and medial plates of pterygoid process
8 Lateral pterygoid muscle
9 Peripharyngeal space
10 Nasopharynx
11 Masseter muscle
12 Levator veli palatini muscle
13 Oropharynx
14 Medial pterygoid muscle
15 Transverse muscle of tongue
16 Soft palate
17 Hypoglossus muscle
18 Mandible
19 Digastric muscle
20 Genioglossus muscle
21 Facial artery
22 Submandibular gland
23 Epiglottic vallecula
24 Hyoid bone (greater horn)
25 Laryngeal vestibule
26 Platysma
27 Piriform recess
28 Aryepiglottic muscle with aryepiglottic fold
29 Omohyoid muscle
30 Thyroid cartilage
31 Thyroarytenoid muscle
32 Arytenoid cartilage
33 Sternocleidomastoid muscle
34 Trachea
35 Anterior jugular vein
36 Thyroid gland
37 Clavicle
38 Inferior thyroid veins

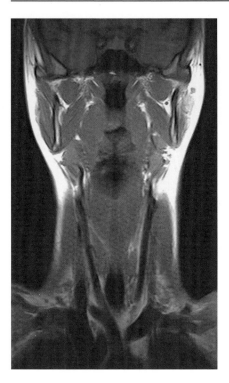

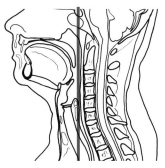

1 Temporal muscle
2 Sphenoidal sinus
3 Sphenoidal bone (greater wing)
4 Oropharynx

5 Zygomatic bone
6 Pharyngotympanic tube (auditory tube)
   (cartilage)
7 Pharyngeal tonsil

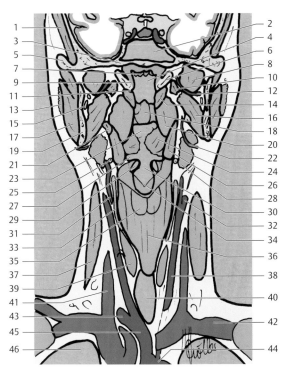

8 Lateral pterygoid muscle
9 Torus tubarius
10 Tensor veli palatini muscle
11 Pharyngeal opening of
   auditory tube
12 Maxillary artery
13 Parotid gland
14 Levator veli palatini muscle
15 Inferior alveolar nerve
16 Medial pterygoid muscle
17 Masseter muscle
18 Soft palate and uvula
19 Ramus of mandible
20 Palatopharyngeus muscle
21 Styloglossus muscle
22 Facial artery
23 Oropharynx
24 Palatine tonsil
25 Hyoid bone
26 Digastric muscle

27 Epiglottic vallecula
28 Submandibular gland
29 Epiglottis
30 Laryngeal inlet
31 External carotid artery
32 Internal carotid artery
33 Thyroid cartilage
34 Interarytenoid notch
35 Posterior cricoarytenoid muscle
36 Middle constrictor muscle of pharynx
37 Sternocleidomastoid muscle
38 Common carotid artery
39 Thyroid gland
40 Trachea
41 Internal jugular vein
42 Subclavian vein
43 Subclavian artery (right)
44 Aorta
45 Brachiocephalic trunk
46 Lung (right)

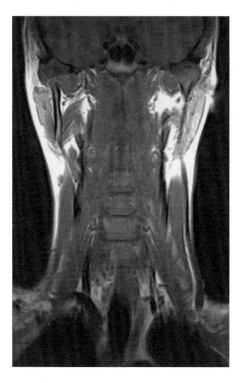

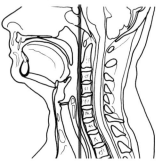

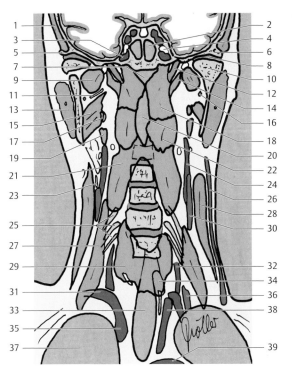

1	Temporal muscle
2	Sphenoidal sinus
3	Internal carotid artery (syphon)
4	Trigeminal cavity
5	Zygomatic process
6	Socket of temporomandibular joint (temporal bone)
7	Nasopharynx
8	Articular disc
9	Lateral pterygoid muscle
10	Head of mandible
11	Lingual nerve
12	Pharyngotympanic tube (auditory tube)
13	Parotid gland
14	Levator veli palatini muscle
15	Medial pterygoid muscle
16	Maxillary artery
17	Stylopharyngeus muscle
18	Longus capitis muscle
19	Digastric muscle
20	Oropharynx
21	Longus colli muscle
22	Longus capitis muscle
23	Vagus nerve (X)
24	Internal carotid artery
25	Spinal nerve roots (cervical plexus)
26	External jugular vein
27	Anterior scalene muscle
28	Sternocleidomastoid muscle
29	Inferior constrictor muscle of pharynx
30	Internal jugular vein
31	Subclavian vein
32	Vertebral artery
33	Trachea
34	Esophagus
35	Brachiocephalic trunk
36	Vertebral vein
37	Lung (right)
38	Common carotid artery
39	Aortic arch

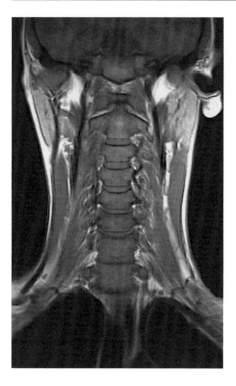

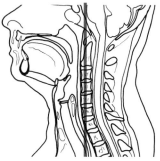

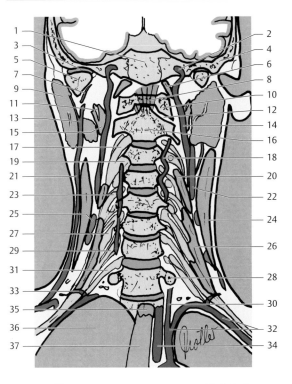

1 Clivus	19 Spinal nerve root C4
2 Internal carotid artery (syphon)	20 Longus colli muscle
3 Articular disc	21 External jugular vein
4 Petrous part of temporal bone	22 Internal jugular vein
5 Head of mandible	23 Spinal nerve root C5
6 Rectus capitis anterior muscle	24 Sternocleidomastoid muscle
7 Maxillary artery	25 Lymph nodes
8 Anterior atlanto-occipital	26 Anterior scalene muscle
membrane	27 Spinal nerve root C6
9 Parotid gland	28 Costal process
10 Atlas (lateral mass)	29 Spinal nerve root C7
11 Styloid process	30 Vertebral artery (left)
12 Atlanto-axial joint	31 Spinal nerve root C8
13 Retromandibular vein	32 Subclavian artery
14 Internal carotid artery	33 Suprascapular artery
15 Digastric muscle	34 Internal carotid artery
16 Axis	35 Esophagus
17 Spinal nerve root C3	36 Lung (right)
18 Vertebral artery	37 Trachea

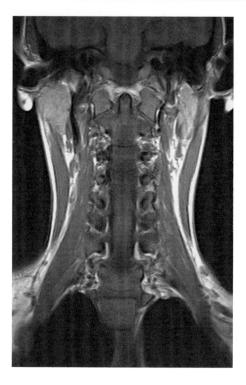

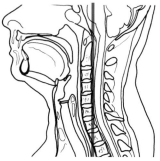

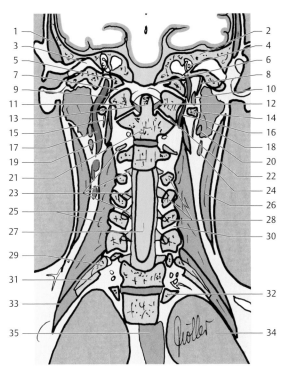

1 Temporal muscle
2 Petrous part of temporal bone
3 External acoustic meatus
4 Tympanic cavity
5 Occipital condyle
6 Clivus
7 Atlanto-occipital joint
8 Styloid process
9 Accessory nerve (XI) and
   hypoglossus nerve (XII)
10 Stylopharyngeus muscle
11 Atlas (lateral mass)
12 Alar ligaments
13 Dens of axis
14 Atlas (transverse process)
15 Vagus nerve (X)
16 Vertebral artery
17 Internal jugular vein
18 Parotid gland
19 Obliquus capitis inferior muscle
20 Stylohyoid muscle
21 Axis (body)
22 Atlanto-axial joint
23 Spinal nerve roots C3–C6
24 Digastric muscle
25 Middle scalene muscle
26 Sternocleidomastoid muscle
27 Spinal cord
28 Articular processes C4–C6
29 Spinal nerve root C8
30 Zygapophysial joint
31 First rib
32 Second rib
33 Posterior scalene muscle
34 Lung (left)
35 Esophagus

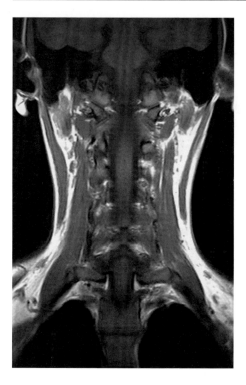

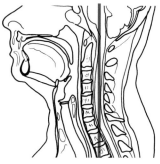

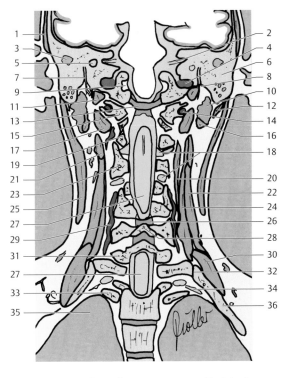

1   Temporal muscle
2   Internal acoustic meatus
3   Mastoid antrum
4   Jugular foramen
5   Vestibule
6   Mastoid process
7   Facial canal
8   Stylomastoid foramen
9   Hypoglossus canal
10 Parotid gland
11 Rectus capitis lateralis muscle
12 Splenius capitis muscle
13 Transverse ligament
14 Vertebral artery
15 Atlas (posterior arch)
16 Digastric muscle (posterior belly)
17 Obliquus capitis inferior muscle
18 Spinal nerve roots
19 Inferior articular process (C2)
20 Spinalis cervicis muscle
21 Longissimus capitis muscle
22 Anterior scalene muscle
23 Superior articular process (C3)
24 Levator scapulae muscle
25 Sternocleidomastoid muscle
26 Ligamentum flavum
27 Spinal cord
28 Arch of C6 vertebra
29 Vertebral artery
30 Scalenus medius muscle
31 Transverse process (C7)
32 Costotransverse joint (T1)
33 Second rib (head)
34 Thoracic nerve (T1)
35 Lung (right)
36 First rib

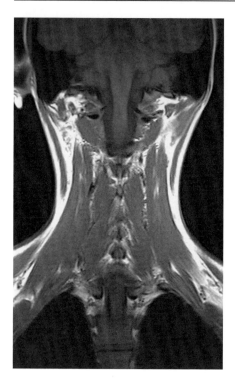

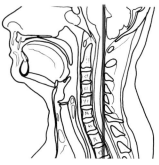

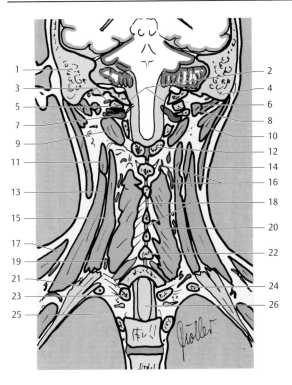

1 Mastoid process (Petrous part of temporal bone)
2 Foramen magnum
3 Suboccipital venous plexus
4 Mastoid process
5 Atlas (posterior arch)
6 Digastric muscle (posterior belly)
7 Vertebral artery
8 Obliquus capitis superior muscle
9 Obliquus capitis inferior muscle
10 Splenius capitis muscle
11 Longissimus capitis muscle
12 Spinous process (C2)
13 Levator scapulae muscle
14 Sternocleidomastoid muscle
15 Splenius cervicis muscle
16 Deep cervical artery and vein
17 Trapezius muscle
18 Interspinous ligaments
19 Deep cervical vein
20 Multifidus muscle
21 Brachial plexus
22 Spinous process (C7)
23 Costal process
24 First rib
25 Lung (right)
26 Spinal cord

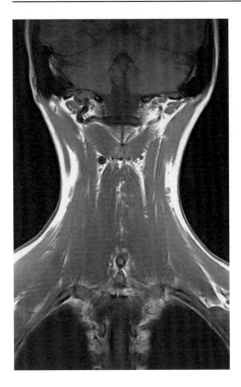

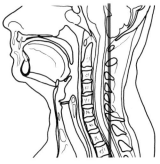

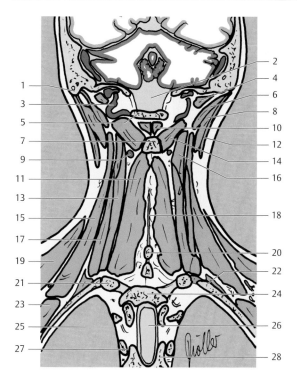

1 Mastoid process
2 Cisterna magna
3 Deep cervical vein
4 Obliquus capitis superior muscle
5 Atlas (posterior arch)
6 Longissimus capitis muscle
7 Spinous process of axis (C2)
8 Splenius capitis muscle
9 Deep cervical vein
10 Rectus capitis posterior major muscle
11 Semispinalis cervicis muscle
12 Sternocleidomastoid muscle
13 Longissimus cervicis muscle
14 Obliquus capitis inferior muscle
15 Levator scapulae muscle
16 Semispinalis capitis muscle
17 Splenius cervicis muscle
18 Supraspinous and interspinous ligaments
19 Trapezius muscle
20 Spinous process (C7)
21 Transverse process (T2)
22 Second rib
23 Supraspinatus muscle
24 Vertebra (T2)
25 Lung (right)
26 Spinal cord
27 Transverse process (T4)
28 Vertebra (T4)

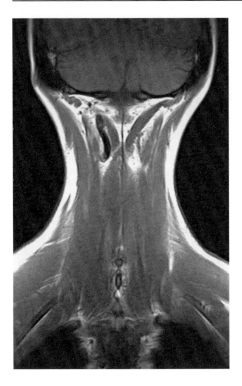

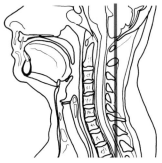

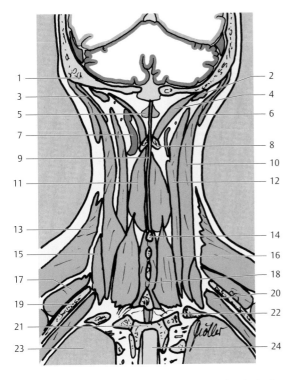

1 Occipital bone
2 Obliquus capitis superior
   muscle
3 Longissimus capitis muscle
4 Rectus capitis posterior major
   muscle
5 Rectus capitis posterior minor
   muscle
6 Sternocleidomastoid muscle
7 Deep cervical vein
8 Spinous process of axis (C2)
9 Nuchal ligament
10 Splenius capitis muscle
11 Semispinalis cervicis muscle
12 Semispinalis capitis muscle
13 Trapezius muscle
14 Spinous process
15 Rhomboid muscle
16 Multifidus muscle
17 Levator scapulae muscle
18 Interspinous ligament
19 Second rib
20 Intercostal muscle
21 Arch of T3 vertebra
22 Costotransverse joint (T3)
23 Lung (right)
24 Spinal cord

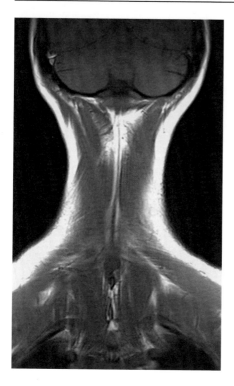

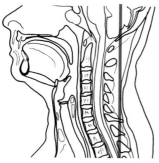

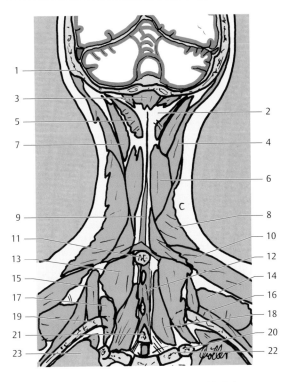

1 Occipital bone
2 Suboccipital fatty tissue
3 Rectus capitis posterior minor
   muscle
4 M. splenius capitis
5 Rectus capitis posterior major
   muscle
6 Semispinalis cervicis muscle
7 Semispinalis capitis muscle
8 Trapezius muscle, descending
   part (superior part)
9 Nuchal ligament
10 Trapezius muscle, transverse
   part (middle part)

11 Spinous process (C7)
12 Interspinous ligament
13 Splenius cervicis muscle
14 Levator scapulae muscle
15 Rhomboid muscle
16 Intercostal muscle
17 Serratus posterior superior muscle
18 Multifidus muscle
19 Third rib
20 Costotransverse joint (T4)
21 Spinous process (T3)
22 Costal process (T4)
23 Lung (right)

Bibliography

Beyer-Enke, S. A., K. Tiedemann, J. Görich, A. Gamroth: Dünnschichtcomputertomographie der Schädelbasis, Radiologie 27 1987: 438–488

Cahill, D. R., M. J. Orland, C. C. Reading: Atlas of Human Cross-Sectional Anatomy. Wiley-Liss, New York 1995

Chacko, A. K., R. W. Katzberg, A. Mac Kay: MRI Atlas of Normal Anatomy. Mc Graw-Hill Inc., New York 1991

Dauber, W.: Pocket Atlas of Human Anatomy, 5th ed. Thieme, Stuttgart 2007 (in print)

El-Khoury, G. Y., R. A. Bergman, E. J. Montgomery: Sectional Anatomy by MRI/CT. Churchill Livingstone, New York 1990

El-Khoury, G. Y., et al.: Essentials in Musculoskeletal Imaging. Churchill Livingstone 2003

Fushimi, Y. et al.: Liliequist Membrane: Three-Dimensional Constructive Interference in Steady State MR Imaging. Radiology 2003: 360–365

Grumme, T., W. Kluge, K. Kretzmar, A. Roesler: Zerebrale und spinale CT. Blackwell, Berlin 1998

Hosten, N., T. Liebig: CT of the Head ans Spine. Thieme, Stuttgart 12002

Huk, W. J., G. Gademann, G. Freidmann: MRI of Central Nervous System Diseases. Springer, Berlin 1990

Kahle, W., M. Frotscher: Color Atlas and Textbook of Human Anatomy, Vol. 3. Thieme, Stuttgart 2003

Kang, M. S., D. Resnick: MRI of the Extremities: An Anatomic Atlas. Saunders, Philadelphia 2002

Koritke, J. G., H. Sick: Atlas of Sectional Human Anatomy. Urban & Schwarzenberg, Baltimore and Munich 1988

Kretschmann, H.-J., W. Weinrich: Cranial Neuroimaging and Clinical Neuroanatomy. Thieme, Stuttgart 2003

Leblanc, A.: Encephalo-Peripheral Nervous System, Springer, Berlin 2001

Meschan, I.: Synopsis of Radiologic Anatomy. Saunders, Philadelphia 1978

Moeller, T. B., E. Reif: MR Atlas of the Musculosketal System. Blackwell Science, Boston 1994

Moeller, T. B., E. Reif: Neuroradiologische Schnittbilddiagnostik. Schnetztor, Konstanz 2002

Moeller, T. B., E. Reif: Pocket Atlas of Radiographic Anatomy, Thieme, Stuttgart 2000

Netter, F. H.: Atlas of Human Anatomy. 4th ed., Saunders, Philadelphia 2006

Rauber, A., Kopsch F.: Anatomie des Menschen. Lehrbuch und Atlas. (eds. H. Leonhardt, Tillmann, G. Töndury, K.Zilles). Vol. I: Bewegungsapparat. Thieme, Stuttgart 2003

Richter, E., T. Feyerabend: Normal Lymph Node Topographie. Springer, Berlin 1991

Rummeny, E. J.: Ganzkörper-MR-Tomographie, 2nd edn. Thieme, Stuttgart 2006

Schnitzlein, H. N., F. Reed Murtagh: Imaging Atlas of the Head and Spine. Urban and Schwarzenberg, Baltimore 1990

Schünke, M. E. Schulte, L. M. Ross, E. D. Lamberti: Thieme Atlas of Anatomy. General Anatomy and Musculoskeletal System. Thieme, Stuttgart 2006

Stark, D. D., W. G. Bradley: Magnetic Resonance Imaging. Mosby, St. Louis 1999

Stoller, D. W., MRI, Arthroscopy, and Surgical Anatomy of the Joints. Lippincott Williams & Willkins, Philadelphia 1999

Stoller, D. W., Tirman, Ph. F. J., Bredella, M. A.: Diagnostic Imaging: Orthopaedics. Amirsys, Salt Lake City, Utah 2004

Uhlenbrock, D.: MR Imaging of the Spine and Spinal Cord. Thieme Stuttgart 2004

Witzig, H.: Punkt-Punkt-Komma-Strich. Falken, Niedernhausen 2000

Index